This work is dedicated to Dr. Pablo Díez and Dr. Patrocinio Morrondo, our mentors at university, and to the whole team of parasitologists from the Faculty of Veterinary of Lugo.

Authors

José Pedreira García
DVM, MS, PhD

Pablo Díaz Fernández
DVM, MS, PhD

María Sol Arias Vázquez
DVM, MS, PhD

Professors of Parasitology and Parasitic Diseases at the Department of Animal Pathology, Faculty of Veterinary Medicine of Lugo, University of Santiago de Compostela, Spain.

1

TABLE OF CONTENTS

Aetiology

Coccidiosis and cryptosporidiosis are the most important parasitic diseases in calves due to their frequency, widespread distribution and clinical significance.

Diarrhoeas of parasitic aetiology in the calf

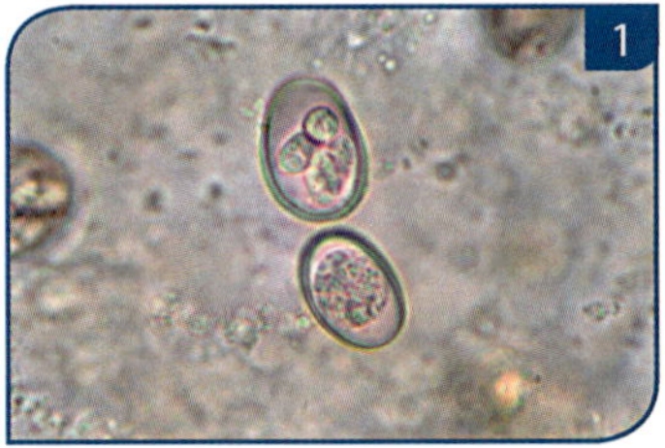

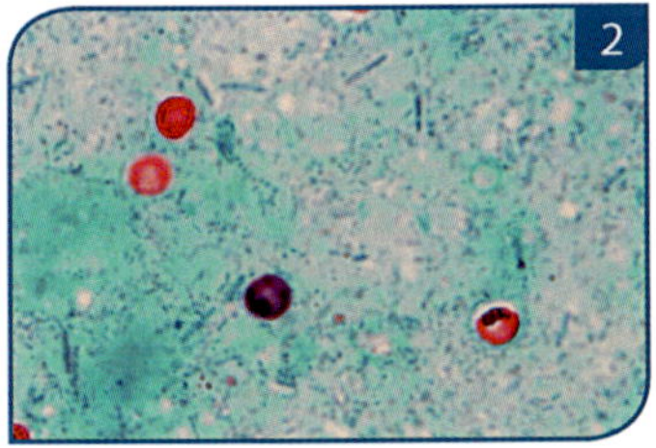

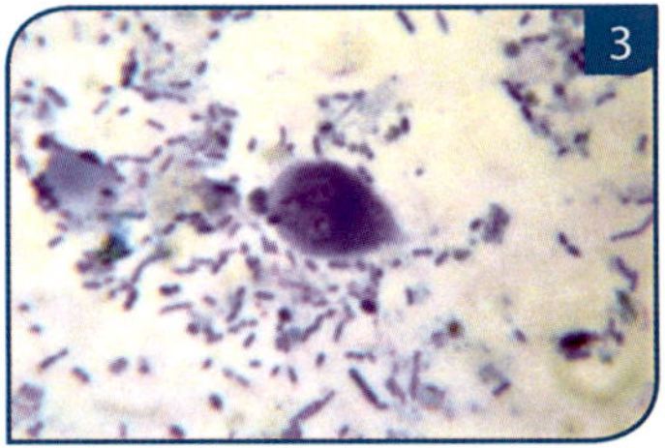

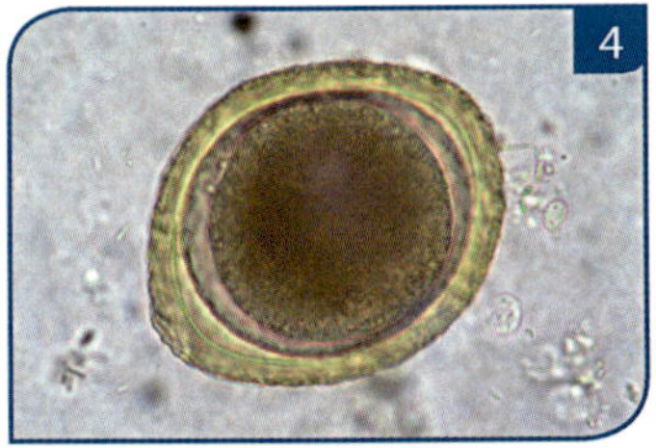

Figure 1. Coccidiosis (*Eimeria bovis, E. zuernii, E. alabamensis*).

Figure 2. Cryptosporidiosis (*Cryptosporidium parvum*).

Figure 3. Giardiasis (*Giardia duodenalis*).

Figure 4. Toxocariasis (*Toxocara vitulorum*).

Biology

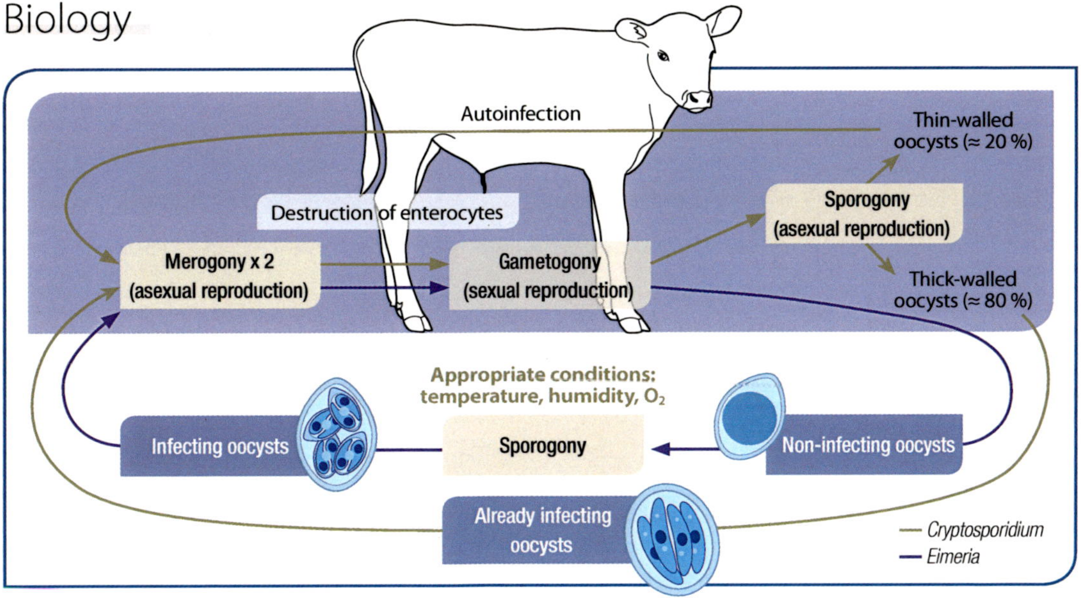

Figure 5. Life cycle of *Cryptosporidium* spp. and *Eimeria* spp.

Epidemiology

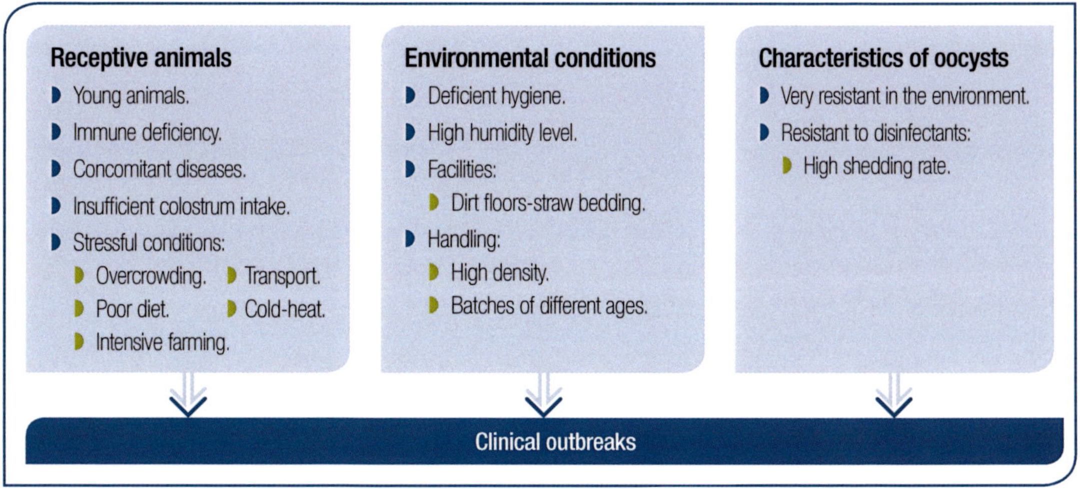

Figure 6. Epidemiological factors favouring the appearance of clinical coccidiosis and cryptosporidiosis in calves.

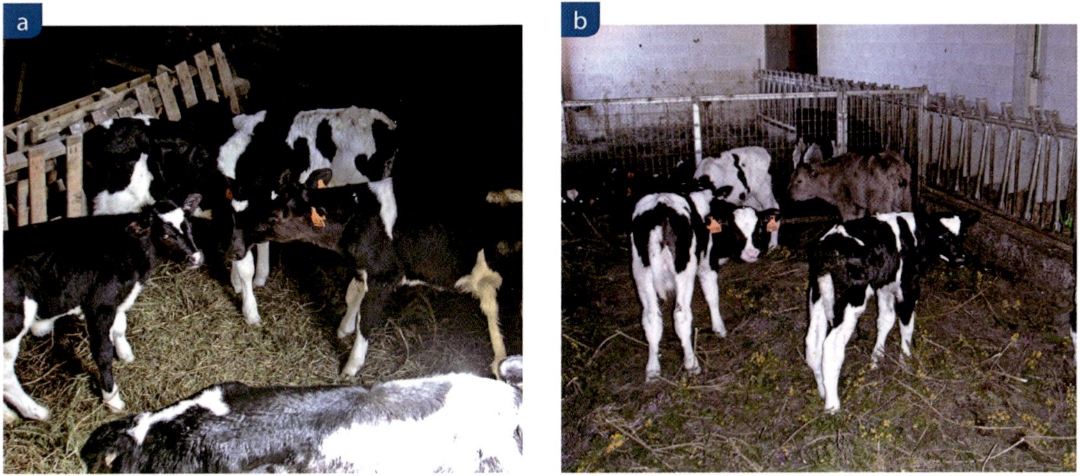

Figure 7. The presence of (a) receptive animals in (b) a very contaminated environment considerably increases the risk of infection and presentation of clinical signs.

Pathogenesis

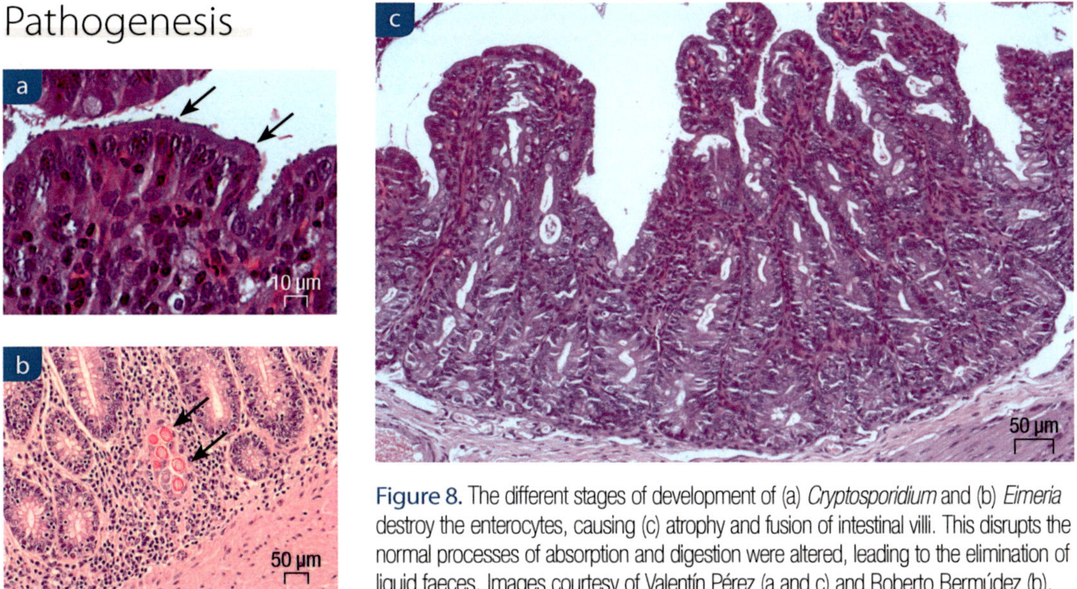

Figure 8. The different stages of development of (a) *Cryptosporidium* and (b) *Eimeria* destroy the enterocytes, causing (c) atrophy and fusion of intestinal villi. This disrupts the normal processes of absorption and digestion were altered, leading to the elimination of liquid faeces. Images courtesy of Valentín Pérez (a and c) and Roberto Bermúdez (b).

Clinical signs

Diarrhoea caused by *Cryptosporidium parvum*:

- Calves <21 days.
- Duration: 3-14 days.
- In the absence of other enteropathogens:
  - Liquid and yellowish faeces.
  - Absence of blood and mucus.

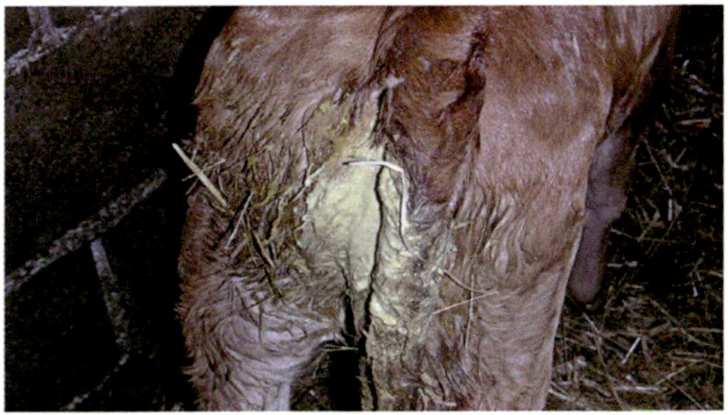

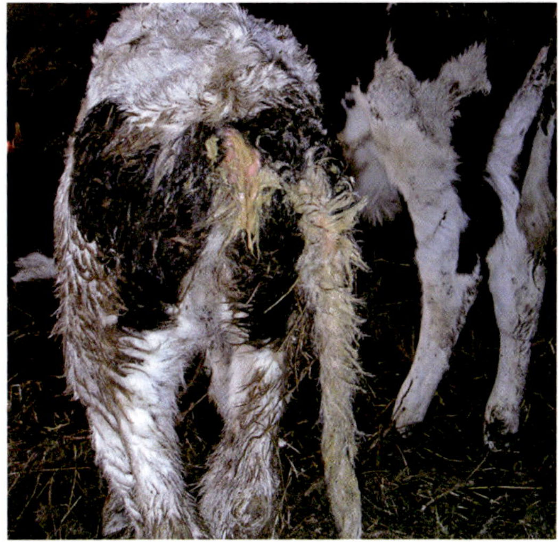

Figure 9. Diarrhoeas caused by *C. parvum* are characterised by the elimination of liquid, yellowish faeces, leaving the calf's tail and hindquarters dirty.

Acute diarrhoea caused by *Eimeria bovis/zuernii*:

- Calves 3 weeks-6 months old.
- Duration: 3-10 days.
- Bloody faeces.
- Presence of mucus, fibrin and tissue remnants.
- Tenesmus.
- Anaemia.

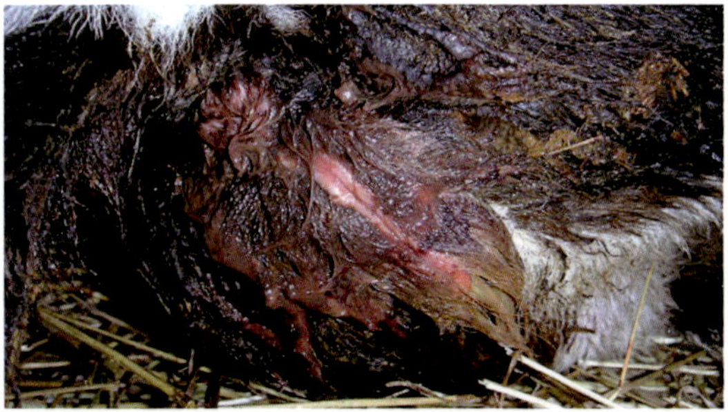

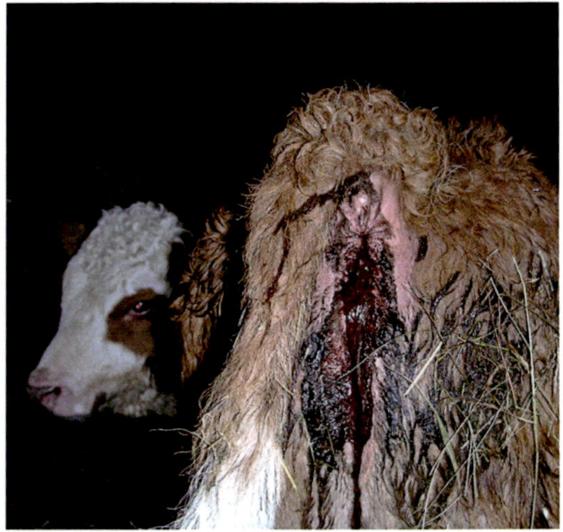

Figure 10. In acute diarrhoeas caused by coccidia, remnants of bloody faeces and mucus are usually observed in the perineal region.

Common clinical signs:

- Apathy.
- Anorexia.
- Dehydration.
- Weight loss.
- Growth delay.
- Susceptibility to other infectious diseases.
- Death.

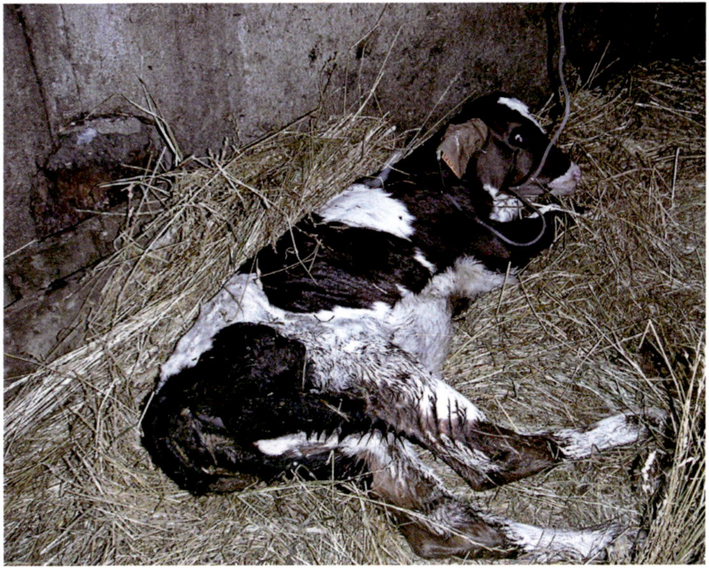

Figure 11. Calves with severe diarrhoea are very weak and need to be rehydrated.

Diagnosis

Faeces

Cryptosporidium

Technique		Characteristics
Staining techniques	Heine	Fast
	Ziehl-Neelsen	Most common
	Auramine	↑ Sensitivity and specificity
Lateral flow test		Fast, easy to read
Direct immunofluorescence		↑ Sensitivity and specificity
Direct ELISA		Many samples processed
PCR		Identification of species

Differential diagnosis:
Rotavirus, Coronavirus, enterotoxigenic *Escherichia coli, Salmonella*

Eimeria

Technique	Characteristics
Flotation	Most common
Sporulation	Identification of species
Scrapings	Absence of oocysts in faeces

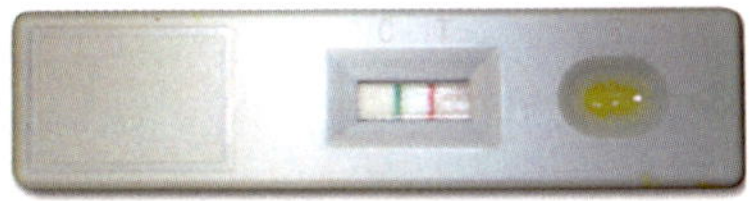

Differential diagnosis:
Gastrointestinal nematodes, *Salmonella*, **BVD**

Figure 12. Most commonly used diagnostic techniques for the detection of *Cryptosporidium* spp. and *Eimeria* spp.

Control

Minimising exposure to new infections

- ↑ Hygiene (cleaning + disinfection)
- ↓ Stress
- Appropriate nutrition

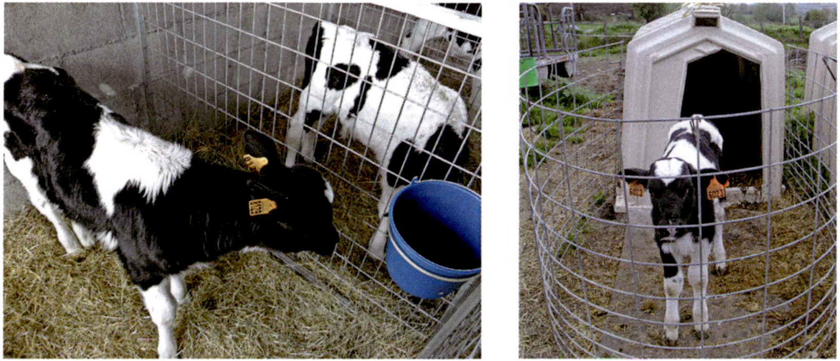

Figure 13. Neonatal diarrhoeas are reduced with careful management and by ensuring maximum hygiene.

Aetiology

- **Ruminal infections**
  Paramphistomum spp.
  Calicophoron spp.
- **Liver infections**
  Fasciola hepatica.
  Dicrocoelium dendriticum.
- **Intestinal infections**
  - **Nematode infections:**
  Trichostrongylid nematodes (*Haemonchus, Ostertagia, Trichostrongylus, Nematodirus, Cooperia*).
  - **Cestode infections:**
  Moniezia spp.

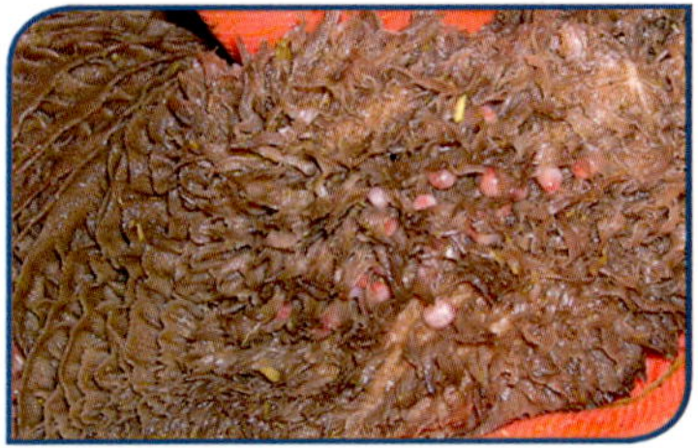

Figure 14. *Paramphistomum* spp. in the ruminal mucosa.

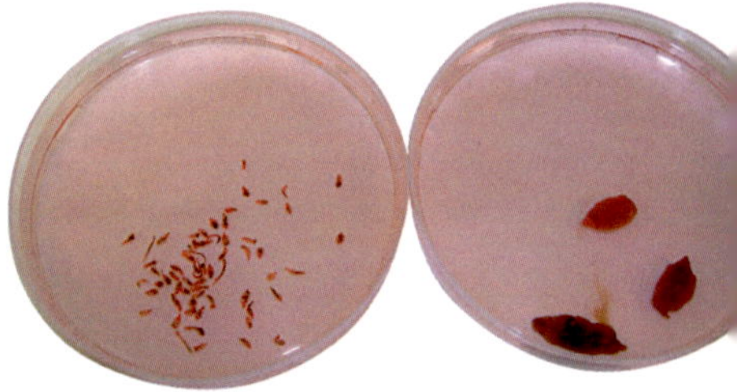

Figure 15. *D. dendriticum* (left) and *F. hepatica* (right) adults.

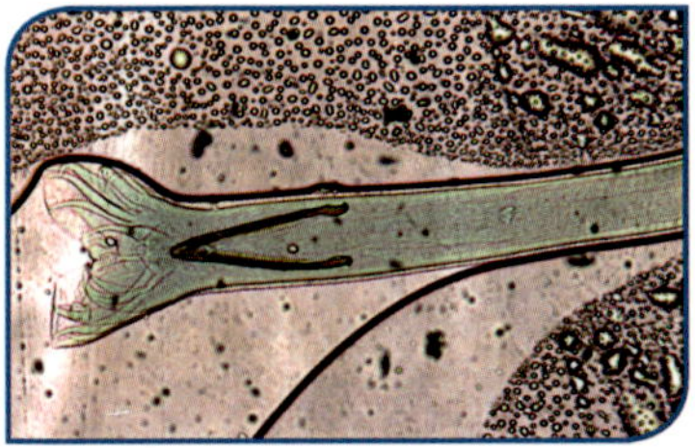

Figure 16. Posterior part of *Haemochus* spp.

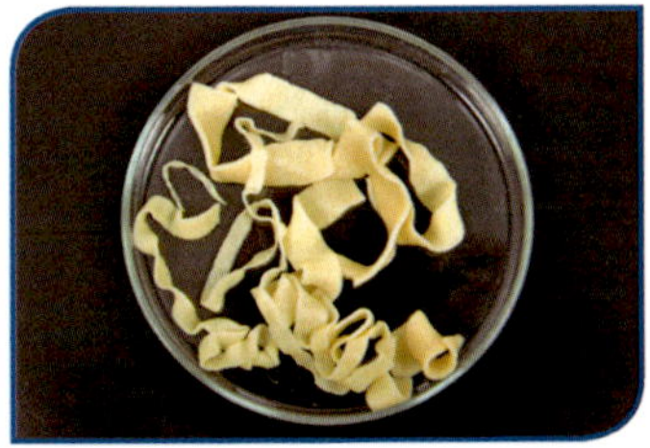

Figure 17. Adult *Moniezia benedeni.*

Biology

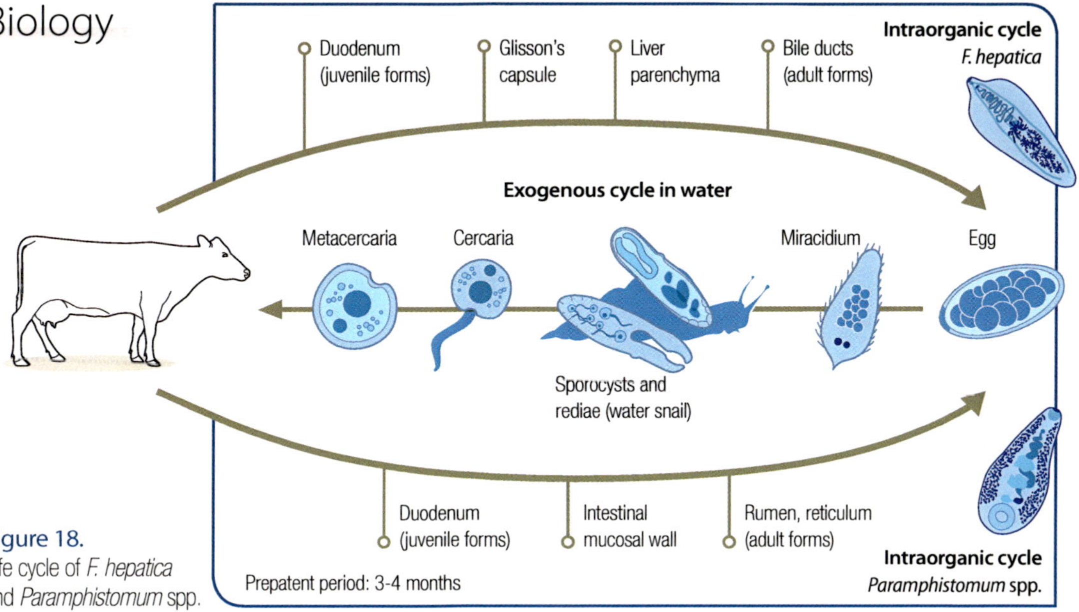

Figure 18. Life cycle of *F. hepatica* and *Paramphistomum* spp.

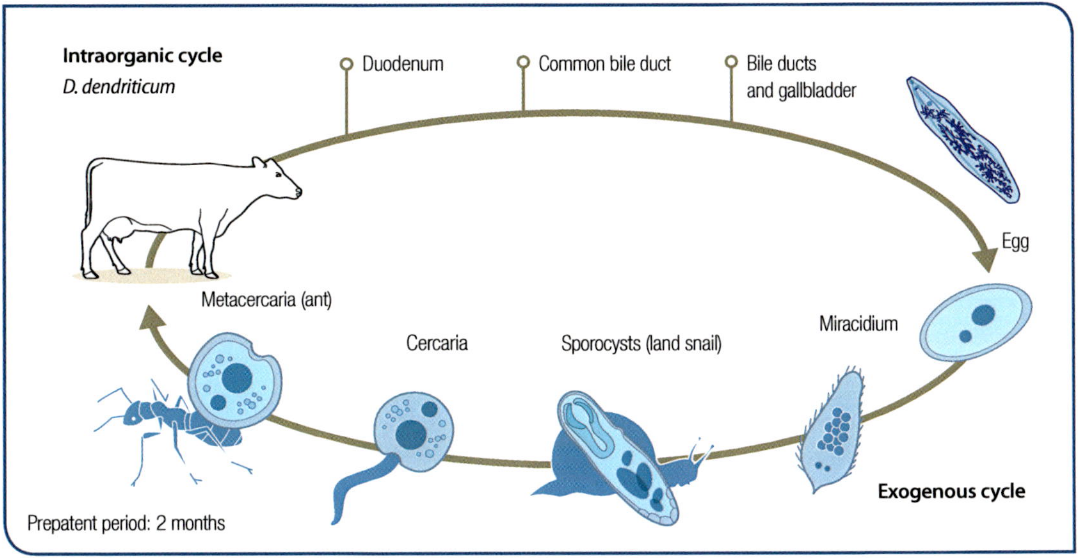

Figure 19. Life cycle of *D. dendriticum*.

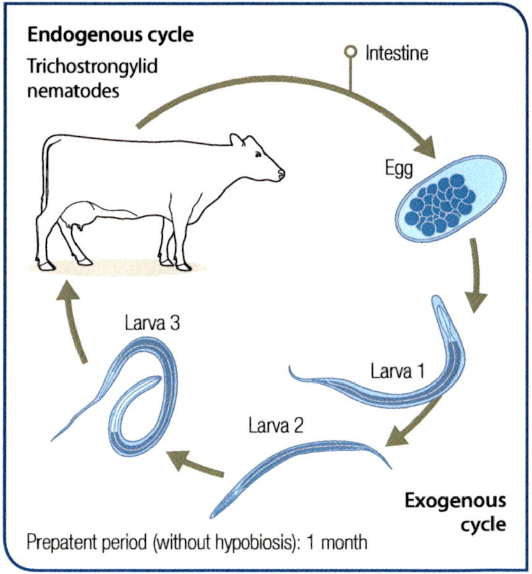

Figure 20. Life cycle of trichostrongylid nematodes.

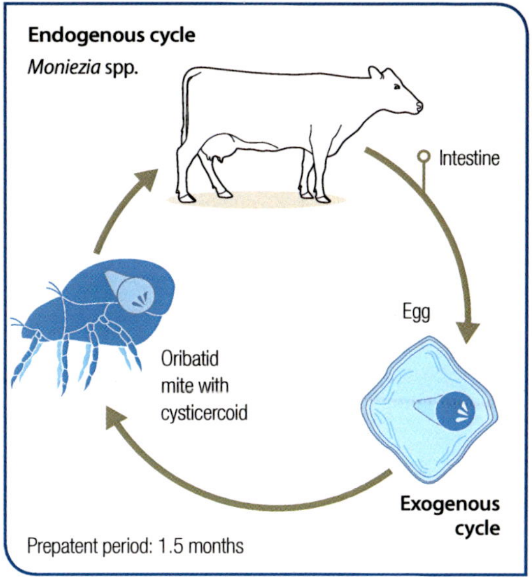

Figure 21. Life cycle of *Moniezia* spp.

Epidemiology

Table 1. Comparative table of the main digestive parasitoses.

	Fasciola hepatica	*Paramphistomum* spp.	*Dicrocoelium dendriticum*	Trichostrongylid nematodes	*Moniezia* spp.
Source of infection	Ingestion of metacercariae attached to the grass or that float in the drinking water		Ingestion of ants with metacercariae	Ingestion of grass with larvae or eggs (*Nematodirus*)	Ingestion of mites with cysticercoids
Intermediate host	Water snails: *Galba truncatula*...		Land snails and ants	–	Oribatid mites
Epidemiology	Grazing in wet pastures with stagnant water, acid soils, mild temperatures		Grazing in dry pastures, limestone soils, sunny weather	Grazing in wet pastures with tall grass. Optimum development >26-27 °C	Grazing in pastures with humus and dense vegetation
Higher risk period	End of spring and autumn		March-November	End of spring and autumn	Rainy seasons

Table 2. Epidemiological characteristics of the main digestive parasitoses.

Parasites	Location	
	Juveniles	Adults
Fasciola hepatica	Liver parenchyma	Bile ducts
***Paramphistomum* spp.**	Small intestine and abomasum	Rumen and reticulum
Dicrocoelium dendriticum	Liver parenchyma	Bile ducts and gallbladder
Trichostrongylid nematodes	-	Abomasum and intestine
***Moniezia* spp.**	-	Small intestine

Clinical signs

Ruminal infections

- Persistent diarrhoea with blood streaks.
- Progressive loss of weight (more obvious in young animals).

Liver infections

- Digestive disorders, especially in younger animals.
- Diarrhoea, ruminal atony, loss of appetite.

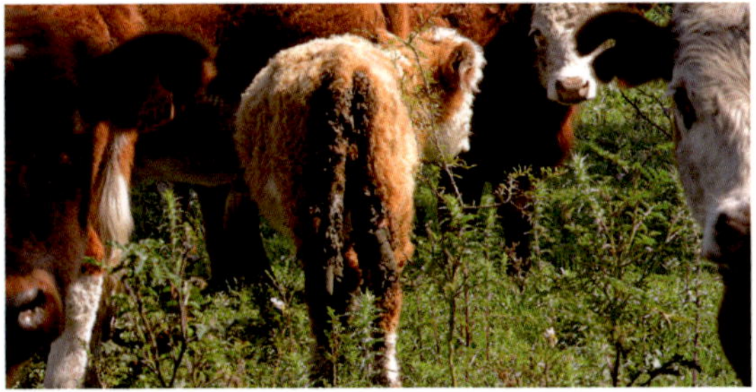

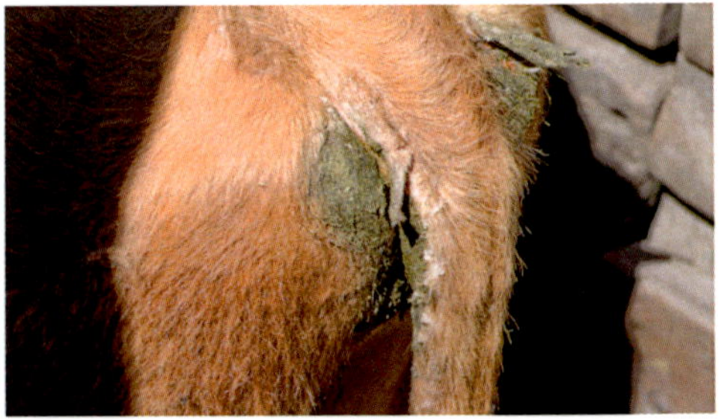

Figure 22. Cattle with profuse diarrhoea caused by trematodes.

Intestinal infections

- **Nematode (roundworm) infections:**
  - Poor general aspect, lack of appetite, diarrhoea.
  - More evident signs during the postpartum period.
- **Cestode infections:**
  - Meteorism.
  - Irregular appetite and rumination.
  - Tenesmus.

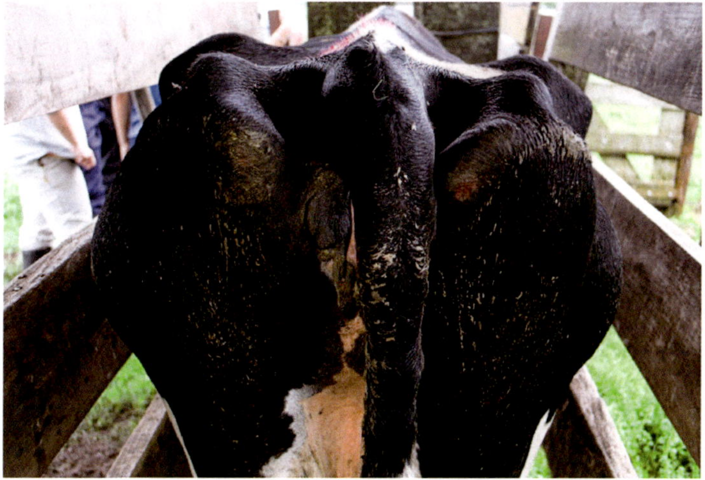

Figure 23. Loss of body condition caused by trichostrongylid nematodes.

Necropsy

Ruminal infections

- Adults attached to the epithelium of the rumen or reticulum.
- Anaemic papillae.
- Areas of necrosis and prominent buttons when parasites detach.
- Calves: juvenile forms in small intestine and abomasum.

Liver infections

- Adults/eggs in bile ducts and gallbladder.
- Fasciolosis:
  - Hypertrophy and brown-yellowish liver.
  - Enlarged and calcified ducts.
  - Enlarged gallbladder and turbid bile.
- *Dicrocoelium* infections:
  - Intense infections: slightly enlarged ducts and enlarged gallbladder.
  - Greenish bile.

Intestinal infections

- **Nematode (roundworm) infections:**
  - Presence of adults and hyperplasia of the mucosa.
  - Nodules and shortening of the villi.
- **Cestode infections:**
  - Adults in small intestine.
  - Obstructions.
  - Erosion and even intestinal perforation (sometimes).
  - Intestinal catarrh, congestive enteritis and oedema.

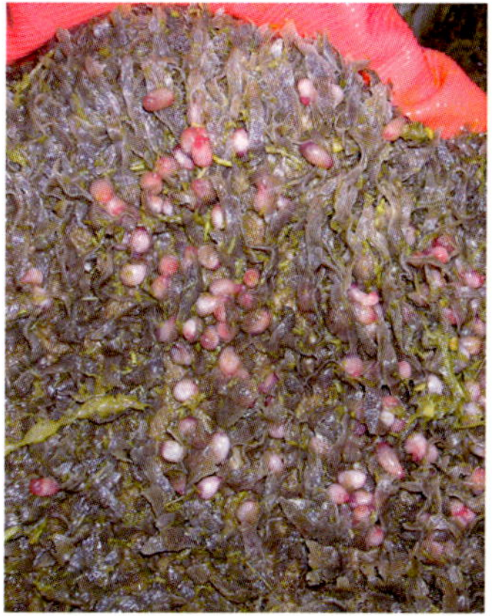

Figure 24. *Calicophoron* adults among the rumen papillae.

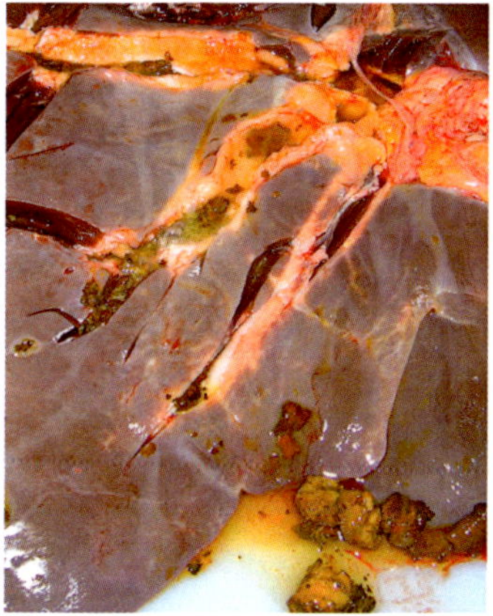

Figure 25. Adult liver flukes (*F. hepatica*) in the hepatic bile canaliculi.

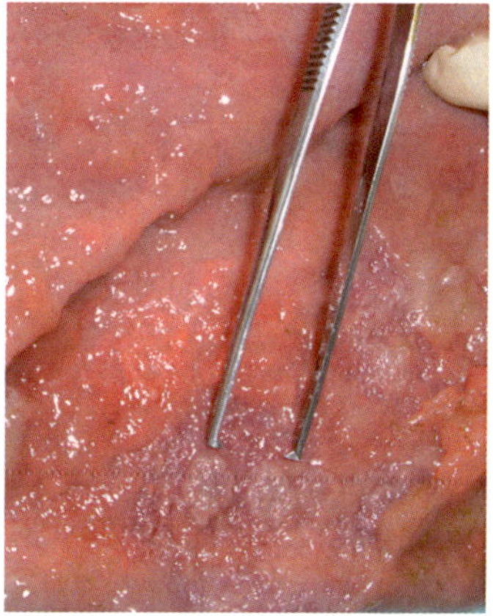

Figure 26. Nodules in the mucosa of the small intestine caused by larvae of trichostrongylid nematodes.

Coprology

Ruminal infections

- Sedimentation.
- False negative results: mild infections in prepatent period.

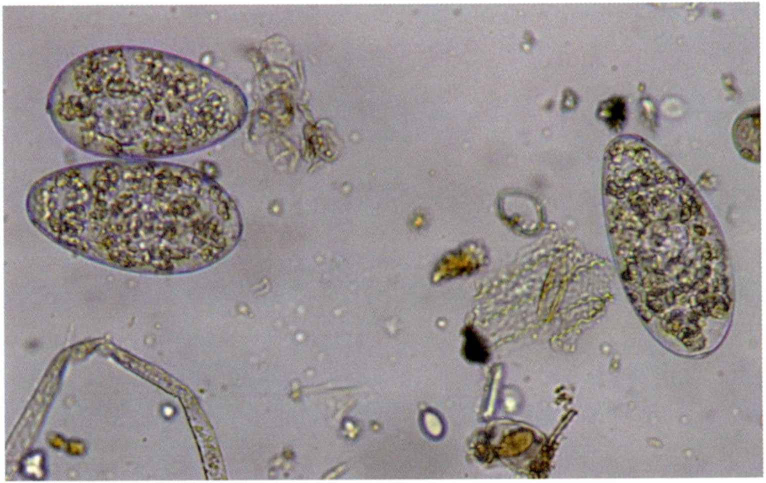

Figure 27.
Eggs of *Calicophoron* spp.

Liver infections

- Sedimentation.
- False negative results: mild infections in prepatent period.

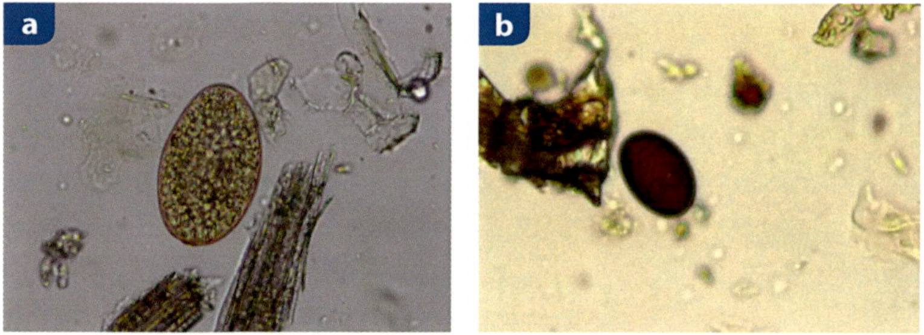

Figure 28. Eggs of (a) *F. hepatica* and (b) *D. dendriticum*.

Intestinal infections

- Faecal flotation.
- False negative results: mild infections in prepatent period.

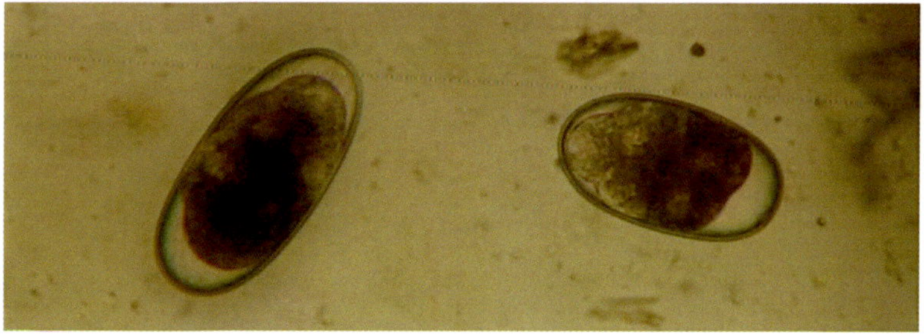

Figure 29. Eggs of trichostrongylid nematodes.

Laboratory

Ruminal infections

- ↓ Red blood cells (RBCs) and haematocrit.
- ↑ Leukocytes and lymphocytes.

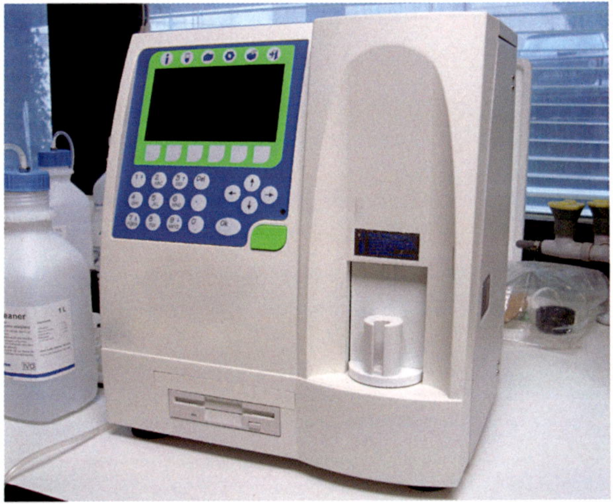

Figure 30. Automated cell counter to quantify blood cell populations.

Liver infections

- Fasciolosis:
  - ↑ GLDH, liver damage.
  - ↑ γ-GT, damage in bile ducts.
  - Anaemia and hypoalbuminaemia.
- *Dicrocoelium* infection:
  - ↑ γ-GT, AST, ALT, LDH and ALP.
  - Eosinophilia and leukocytosis.

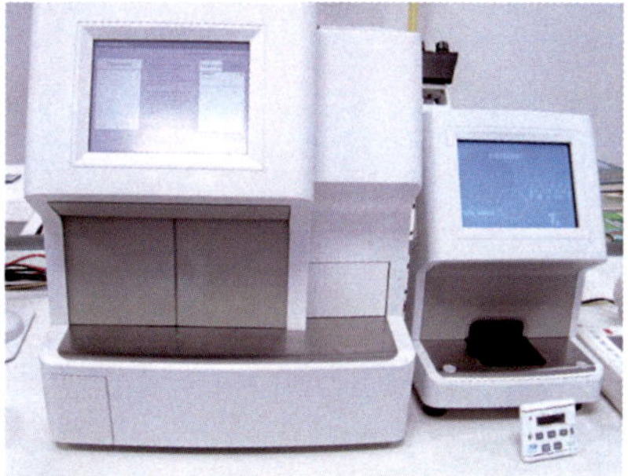

Figure 31. Spectrophotometer to measure enzymatic activity.

Intestinal infections

Trichostrongylid nematodes:
↑ serum pepsinogen concentration.

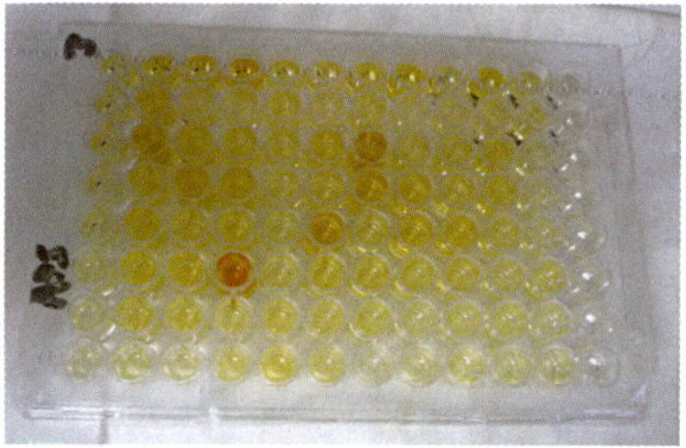

Figure 32. Determination of serum pepsinogen using microtitre plates.

Preventive measures

Ruminal infections

- Fencing in swamp areas.
- Draining pasture lands.
- Elevated drinking troughs.
- Manure fermentation.
- Drying hay and good-quality silage.
- Draining pasture fields.

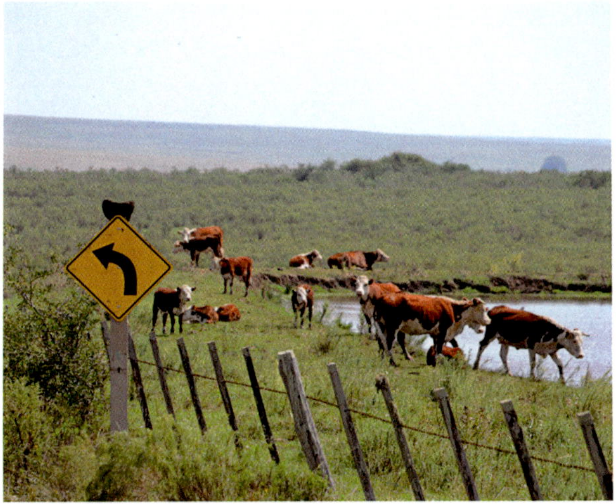

Figure 33. Grazing in wet areas favours infection by trematodes.

Liver infections

- Fasciolosis:
  - Same measures as for paramphistome infections.
- *Dicrocoelium* infections:
  - Avoid grazing early in the morning and in the evening.

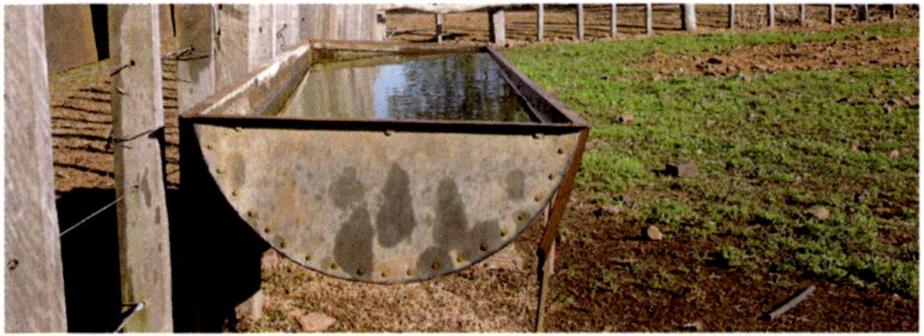

Figure 34. Placing drinking troughs in elevated locations reduces the risk of parasitation by trematodes.

Intestinal infections

- Fields left fallow and cultivated.
- Alternate grazing with different species.
- Grazing with animals of different ages.
- Cestode infections: avoid grazing early in the morning and in the evening.

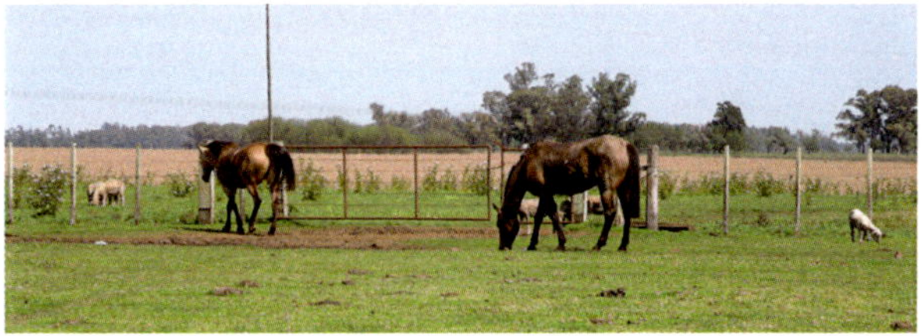

Figure 35. Mixed grazing with different species may favour infection by trichostrongylid nematodes.

Biological control

Ruminal and liver infections

- Harmless saprophytic fungi.
- Marked **ovicidal effect.**
- Hyphae of fungi grow in the presence of parasite eggs; they penetrate through the egg-shells and destroy them.

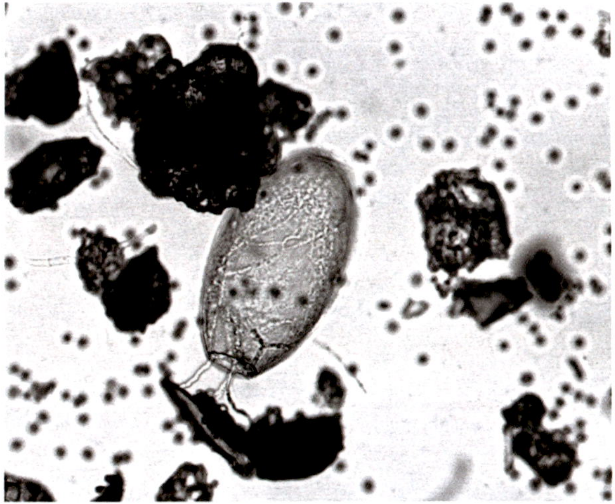

Figure 36. Action of ovicidal fungi on tremadote eggs.

Intestinal infections

- Harmless saprophytic fungi.
- Marked **ovicidal effect.**
- The fungi form webs of hyphae and rings in which the larvae of different gastrointestinal strongyle nematodes are retained.

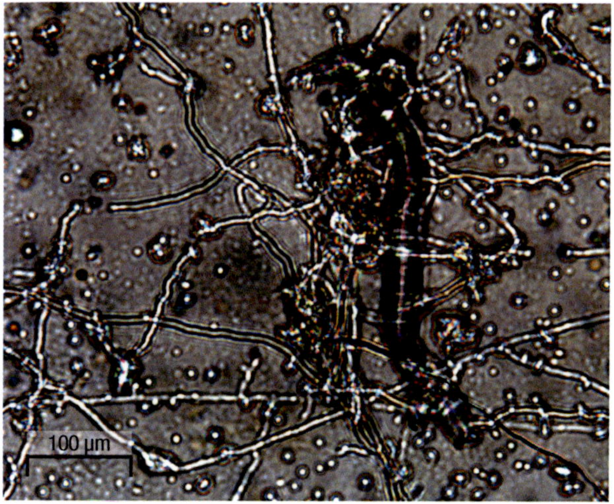

Figure 37. Fungi developing traps with which they catch nematode larvae.

Aetiology

In the Northern Hemisphere, babesiosis and theileriosis are the most important blood parasitic infections due to their frequency, wide distribution and clinical significance.

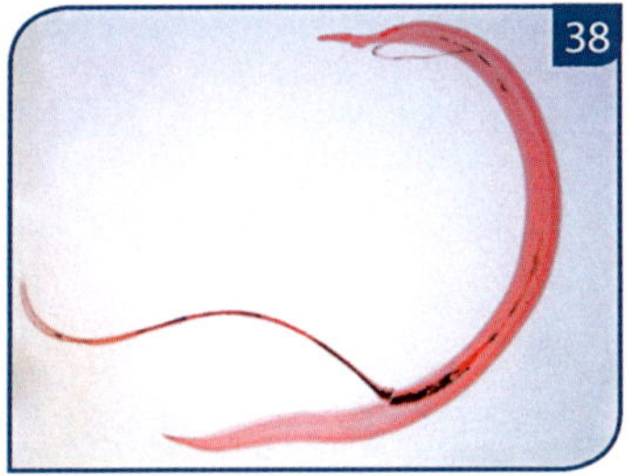

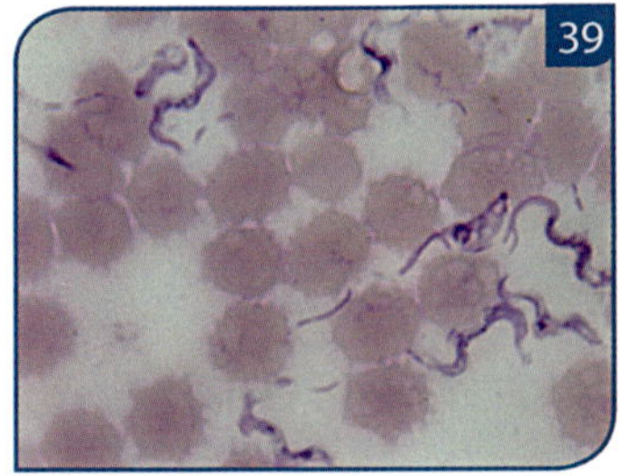

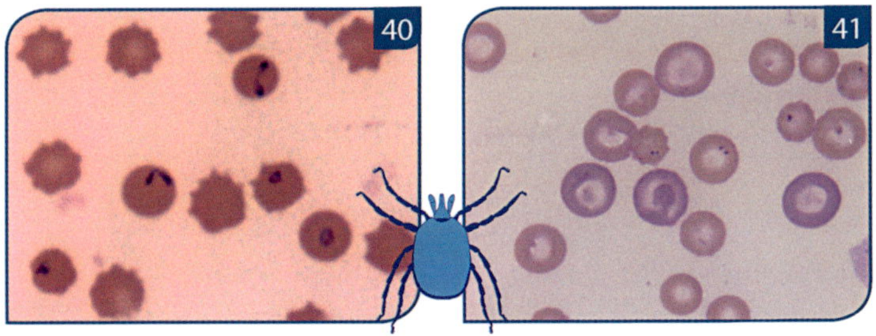

Figure 38. Schistosomiasis (*Schistosoma* spp.).

Figure 39. Trypanosomiasis (*Trypanosoma* spp.).

Figure 40. Babesiosis (*Babesia bovis, B. bigemina, B. divergens, B. major).*

Figure 41. Theileriosis (*Theileria* spp.).

Biology

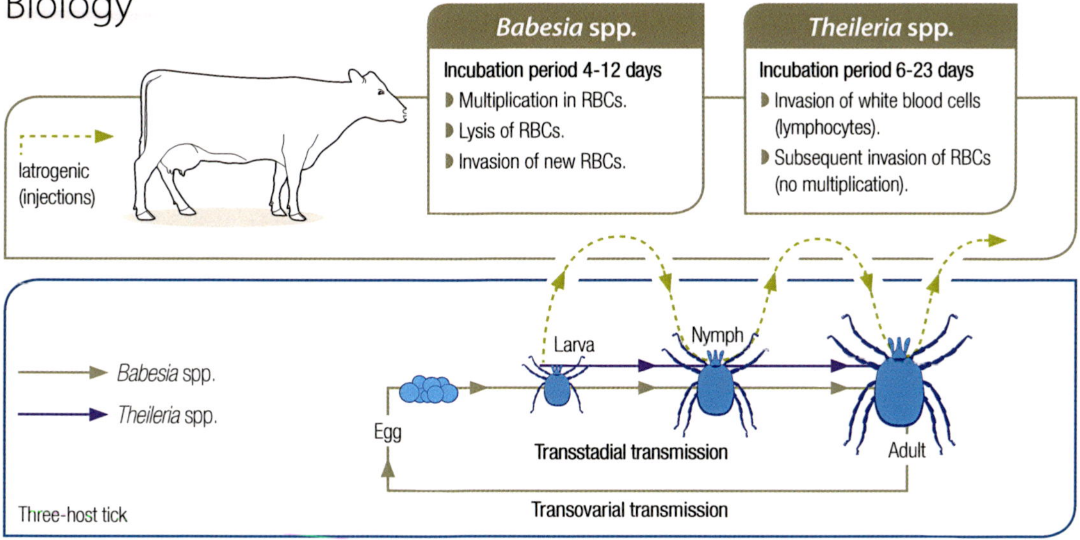

Figure 42. Life cycle of *Babesia* spp. and *Theileria* spp.

Epidemiology

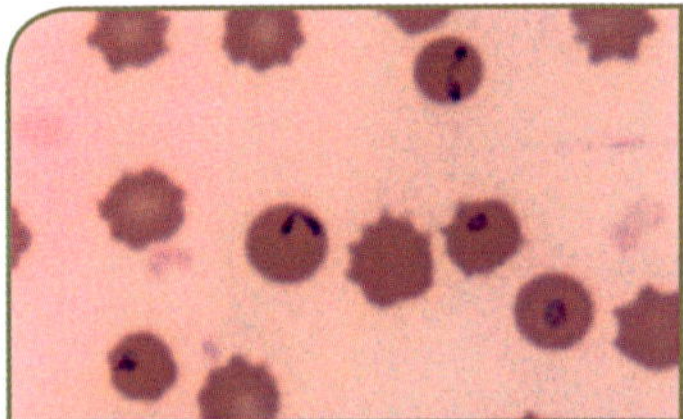
Babesia divergens

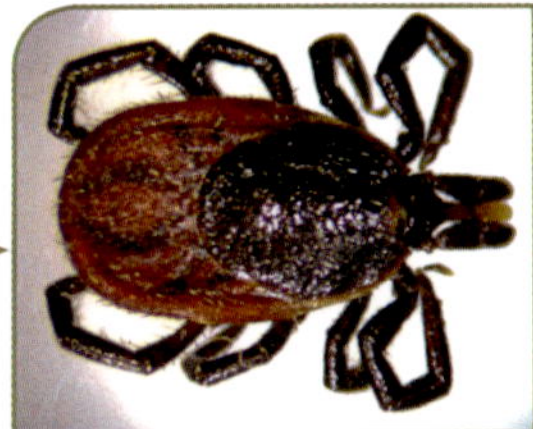
Ixodes ricinus

- Less severe clinical pictures.
- Mortality only in severe clinical pictures.
- Zoonotic potential.

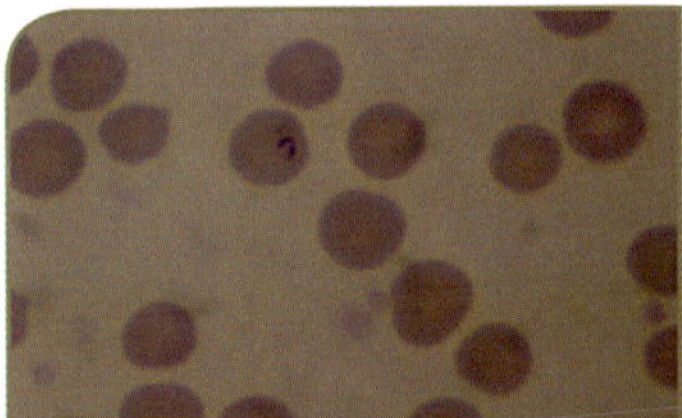
Babesia bovis

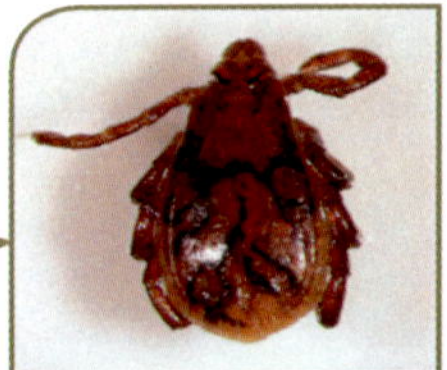
Rhipicephalus annulatus

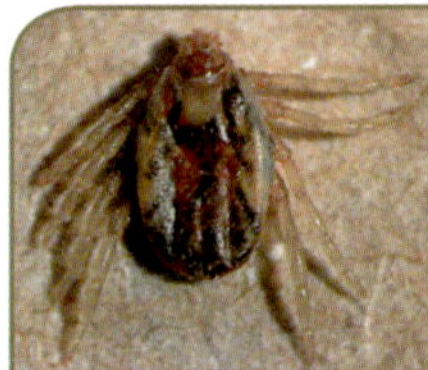
* *Rhipicephalus (Boophilus) microplus*

- Very virulent.
- 70-80 % mortality without treatment.

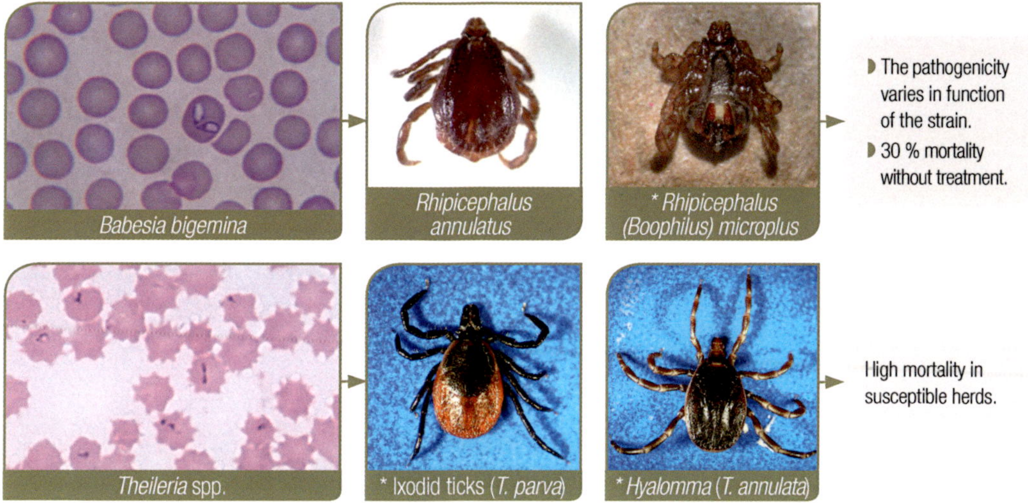

Figure 43. Characteristics of piroplasms affecting cattle. * Images courtesy of José Manuel Venzal.

Clinical signs

Babesiosis

- Fever (parasitaemia)
- **Anaemia**
- Jaundice
- Lack of energy
- Abortions
- Agalactia
- Slow recovery
- **Haematuria**

Acute or cerebral form

- Ataxia
- Pedalling movements
- Haemolysis
- Jaundice
- Haematuria

(Haemolysis, Jaundice, Haematuria: Not noticeable in the early stages)

Theileriosis

- Similar to babesiosis
- **Higher fevers (up to 42 °C)**
- Dyspnoea
- **Significant lymph node infarction**
- Haemoglobinuria (not always)
- Dark faeces or with clotted blood

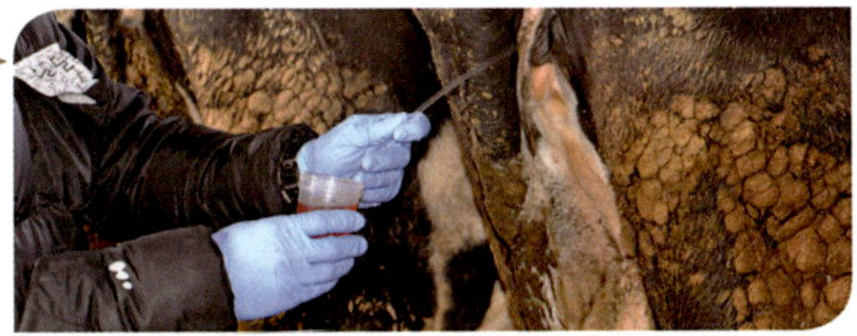

Figure 44. Main clinical signs of bovine piroplasmosis.

Diagnosis

Clinical suspicion
Clinical signs associated with haemolysis and haemoglobinuria
- Presence of ticks on the animal.

Confirmation. Laboratory diagnosis
Collection of whole blood (EDTA)/serum

Microscopic techniques
Observation of intraerythrocytic forms
- Thin blood smear.
- Low sensitivity.
- Experienced workers.
- Lymph node imprint cytology (*Theileria*).

Molecular techniques
Detection of parasite DNA
- PCR test from blood or ticks.

Immunological techniques
Antibody detection in serum
- ELISA.
- Indirect immunofluorescence (IIF).
- See availability.

Figure 45. Main techniques for the diagnosis of piroplasmosis in ruminants.

Differential diagnosis

Anaplasmosis, trypanosomiasis, leptospirosis, etc.

Prevention and control

Eliminating/reducing the presence of the invertebrate vector to prevent the appearance of new cases.

Aetiology

Main parasites affecting reproductive system in cattle

Neospora caninum is the parasite with greatest impact on reproduction in cattle.

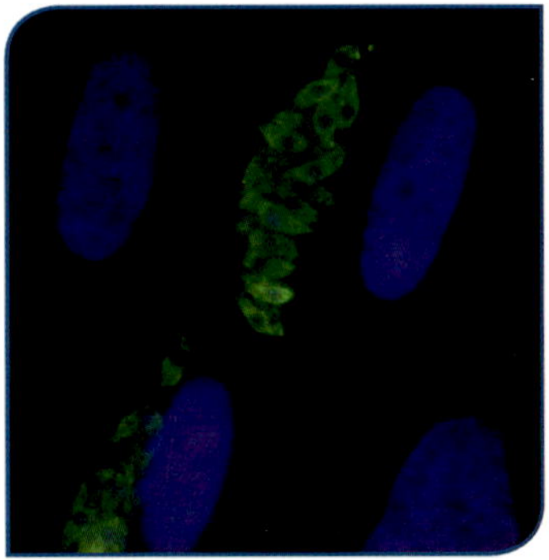

Figure 46. Cell culture of *N. caninum*.

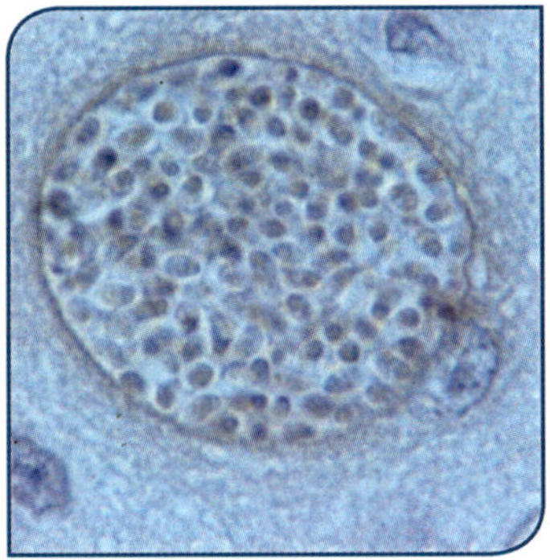

Figure 47. *T. gondii* cyst.

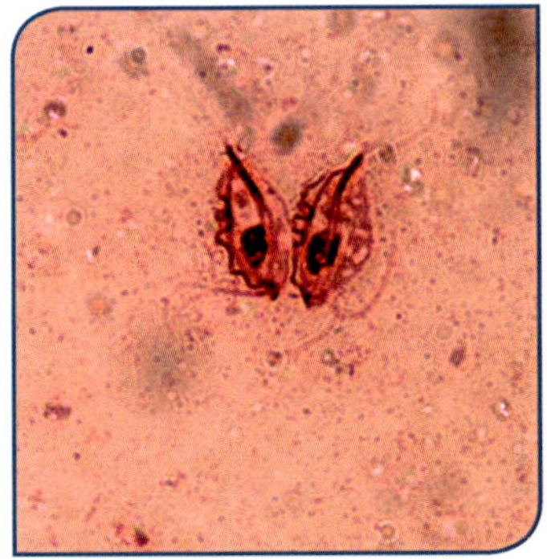

Figure 48. *T. foetus* trophozoites.

Images courtesy of SALUVET Group, Complutense University of Madrid.

Biology

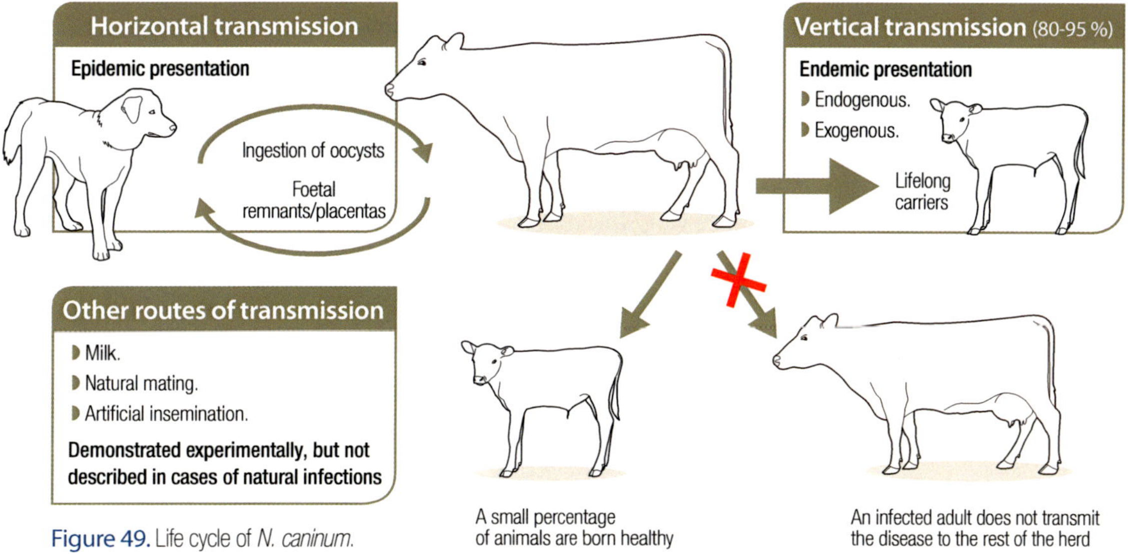

Figure 49. Life cycle of *N. caninum*.

Pathogenesis and clinical signs

The multiplication of *Neospora caninum* creates necrotic foci with a non-purulent inflammatory response (predilection for CNS, muscle tissue and endothelium).

1st third

- Embryonic resorption.
- New oestrus.

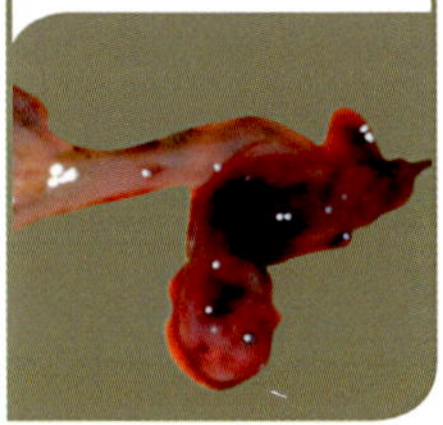

2nd third

- **Abortions.**
- Mummified foetuses.

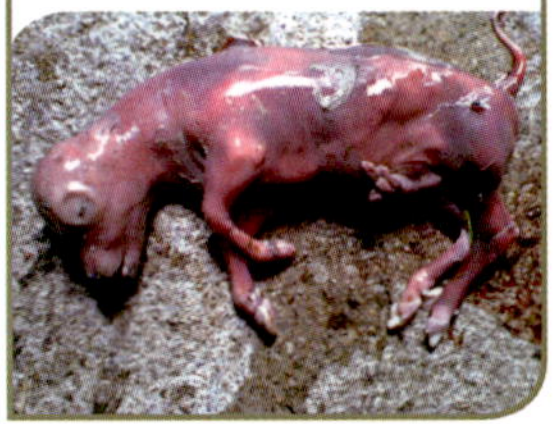

Final third

- **90-95 % of healthy animals infected by congenital route.**
- Weak animals with nervous problems and perinatal mortality.

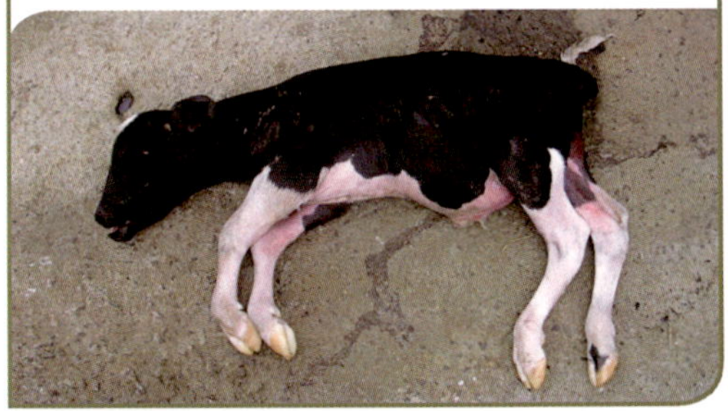

Figure 50. The clinical signs vary depending on the time when the foetus is infected.

Clinical signs in the infected calf:

- Birth of a weak or even normal animal.
- Neuromuscular symptoms:
  - Extended limbs.
  - Lack of coordination.
  - Ataxia.
  - Ocular asymmetry.
  - Malformations.

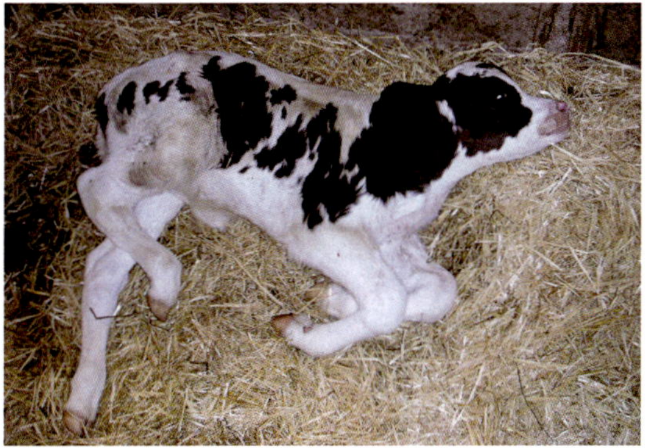

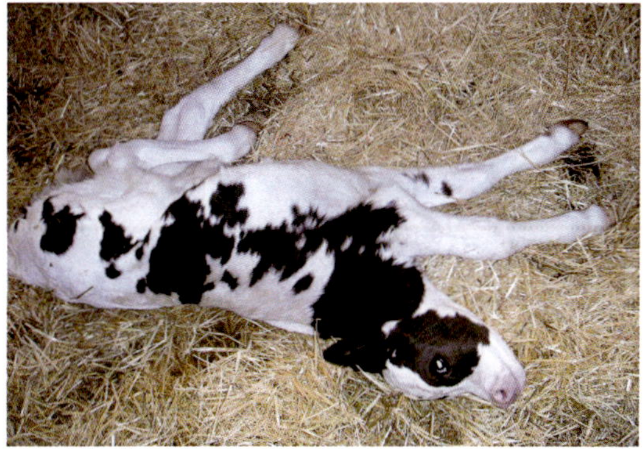

Figure 51. Weak calves born from cows positive to *Neospora*.

Diagnosis

- Based on laboratory confirmation after a suspicion due to the appearance of abortions.
- Detection of antibodies in blood (mother/foetus) or foetal fluids: IFA, indirect ELISA, Western blot.
- In foetal tissues (brain, spinal cord and heart):
  - Histology: compatible lesions.
  - Immunohistochemistry.
- Molecular biology tests: PCR.
- Bulk tank tests to monitor the herd are available.

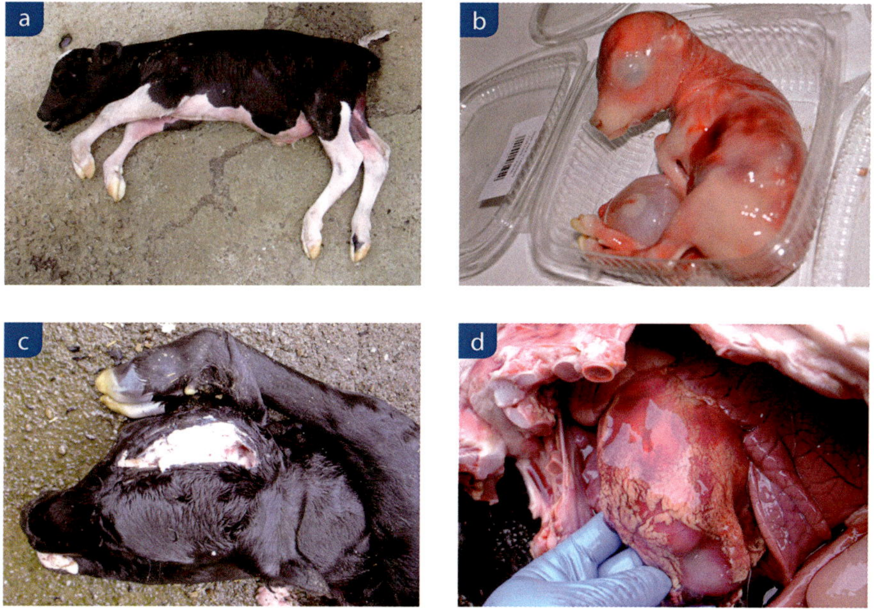

Figure 52. In cases of (a) abortions, it is recommended to submit (b) the foetus, placenta and foetal fluids to the laboratory and, if this is not possible because of their size, to collect samples from the (c) brain and (d) heart.

Control

Preventing new infections (horizontal transmission)

- Prevent dogs and hosts from gaining access to the premises.
- Clean drinking and feeding troughs regularly.
- Destroy aborted foetuses and placentas.
- Analyse newly arrived animals.

Avoiding their spread (vertical transmission)

- Accelerate the replacement of positive animals.
- Do not breed from seropositive cows.
- Check breeding procedures and bulls.

The use of beef bulls in seropositive Holstein cows reduces the percentage of abortions. In addition, breeding from their offspring should be avoided.

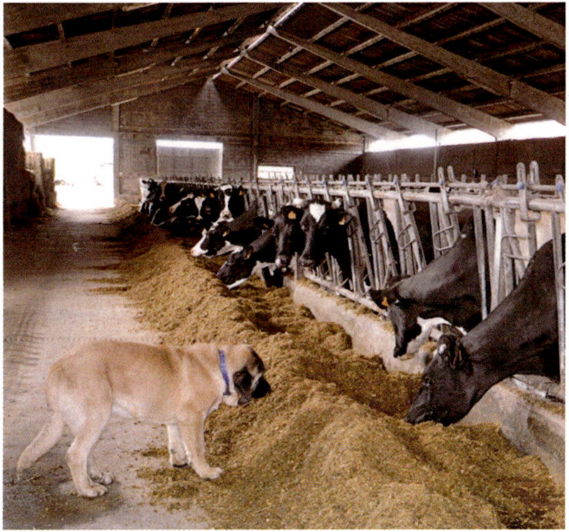

Figure 53. Dog with access to the cows' feeding troughs.

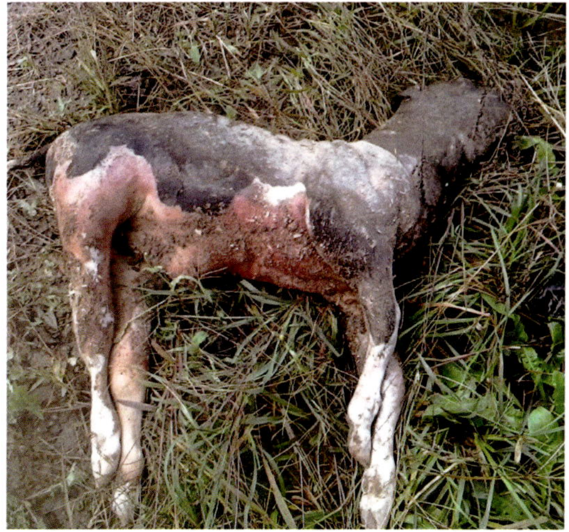

Figure 54. Inappropriate management of an abortion.

Aetiology

Main parasites responsible for skin disorders in cattle

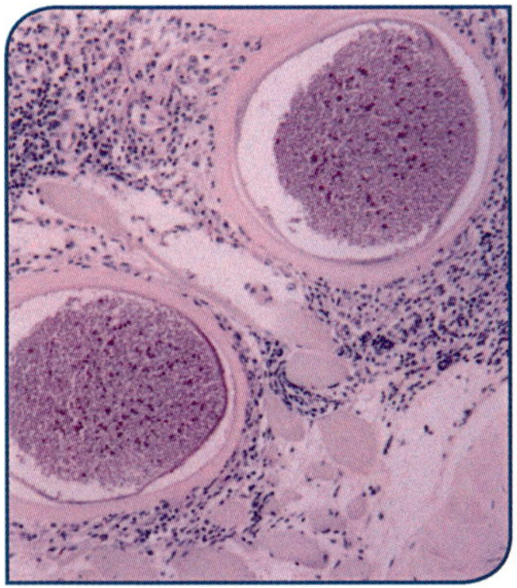

Figure 55. Besnoitiosis (*Besnoitia besnoiti*).

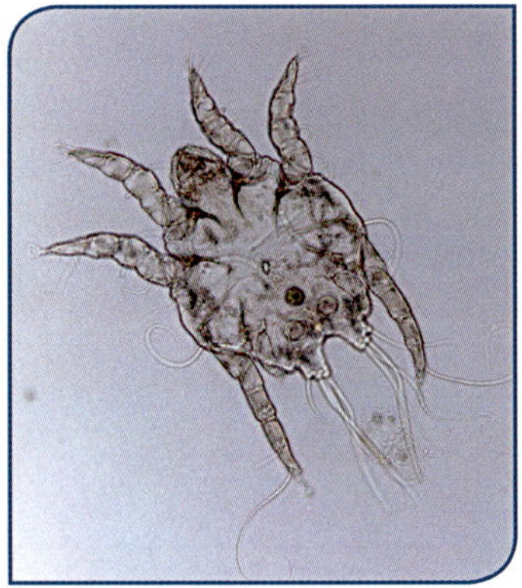

Figure 56. Mange (*Sarcoptes*, *Psoroptes*, *Chorioptes*, etc.).

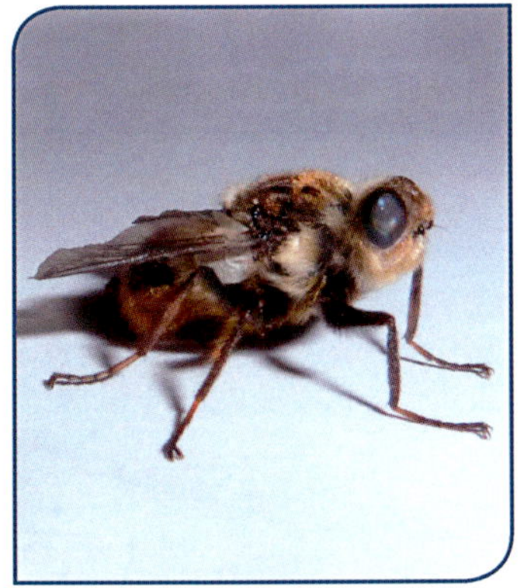

Figure 57. Hypodermosis (*Hypoderma bovis*, *Hypoderma lineatum*).

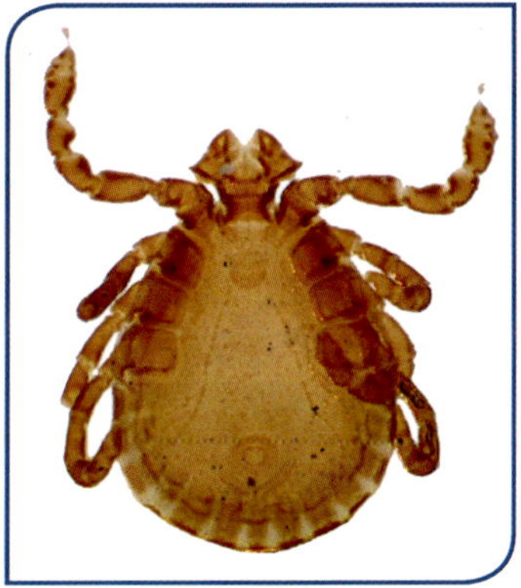

Figure 58. Infections caused by ticks (*Ixodes*, *Haemaphysalis*, *Rhipicephalus*, etc.).

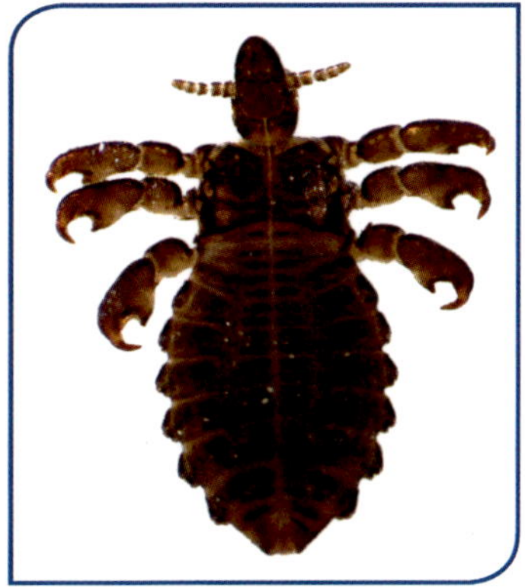

Figure 59. Pediculosis (*Bovicola*, *Haematopinus*, *Linognathus*, etc.).

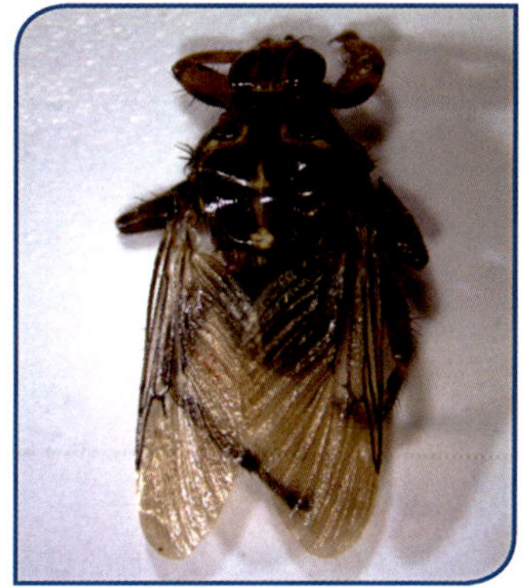

Figure 60. Other parasites (*Stephanofilaria stilesi*, *Hyppobosca equina*, horseflies, flies).

Hypodermosis

Biology

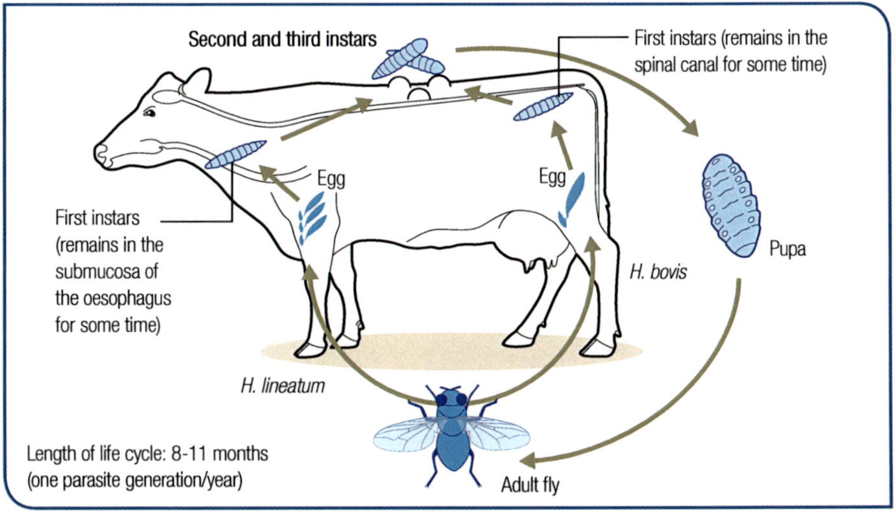

Figure 61. Life cycle of *H. bovis* and *H. lineatum.*

Clinical signs

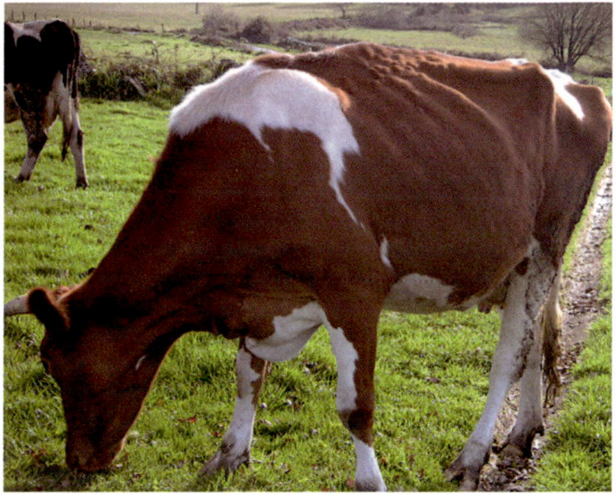

Economic losses:

- ↓ Milk production.
- ↓ Growth.
- ↓ Carcass quality.
- Self-injury (escape response).
- Secondary infections/myiases.

Figure 62. Lumps of larvae or warbles on the back of a cow.

Lesions

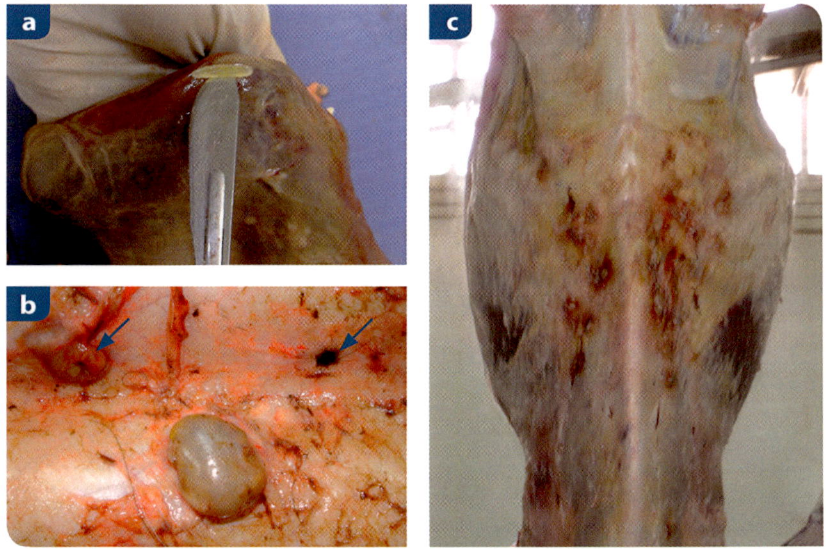

Figure 63. (a) Stage I larvae of *H. lineatum* in the submucosa of the oesophagus. (b) Stage II and III larvae, in the interior of the warbles, perforate the skin (arrow) and (c) damage the subcutaneous tissue. Images courtesy of Dr. Rosario Panadero.

Diagnosis and control

	Early (autumn)	**Late (spring)**
Diagnosis	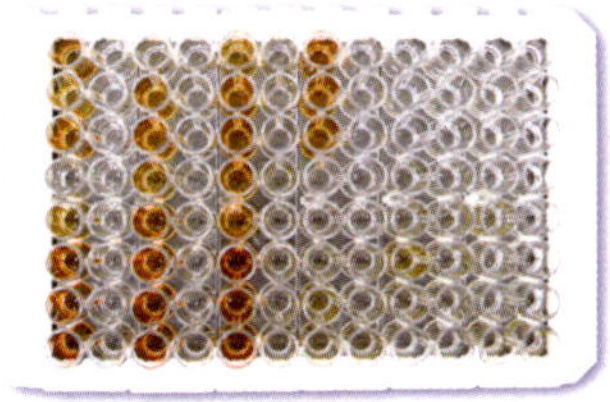 Immunoenzymatic techniques (ELISA)	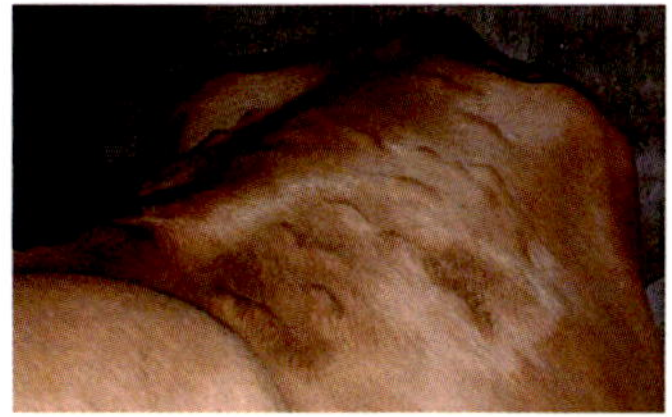 Counting warbles on the animal's back
Treatment	◗ Eliminates migrating stage I larvae. ◗ After the end of the fly season. ◗ Prevents most significant damage. ◗ **Possible adverse effects!** Very late treatments (>November).	◗ Against stage II and III larvae on the back. ◗ Does not prevent most significant damage. ◗ Controls the fly population and possible reinfections.

Figure 64. Times to make a diagnosis and treat hypodermosis.

Tick infestation

Aetiology

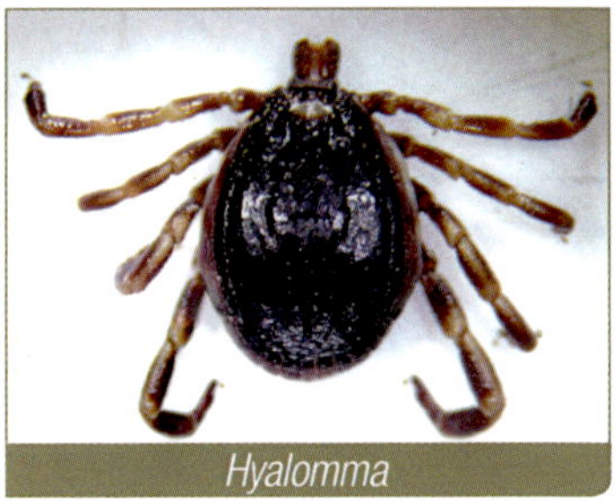

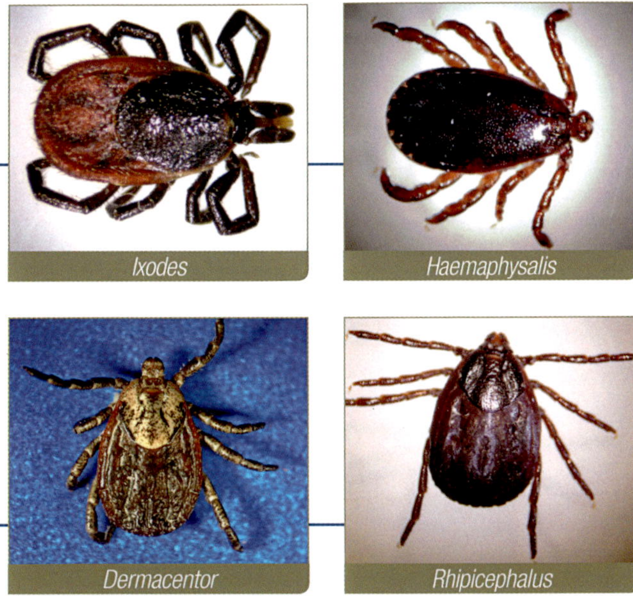

Figure 65. Genera of the most common hard ticks in Europe.

Biology

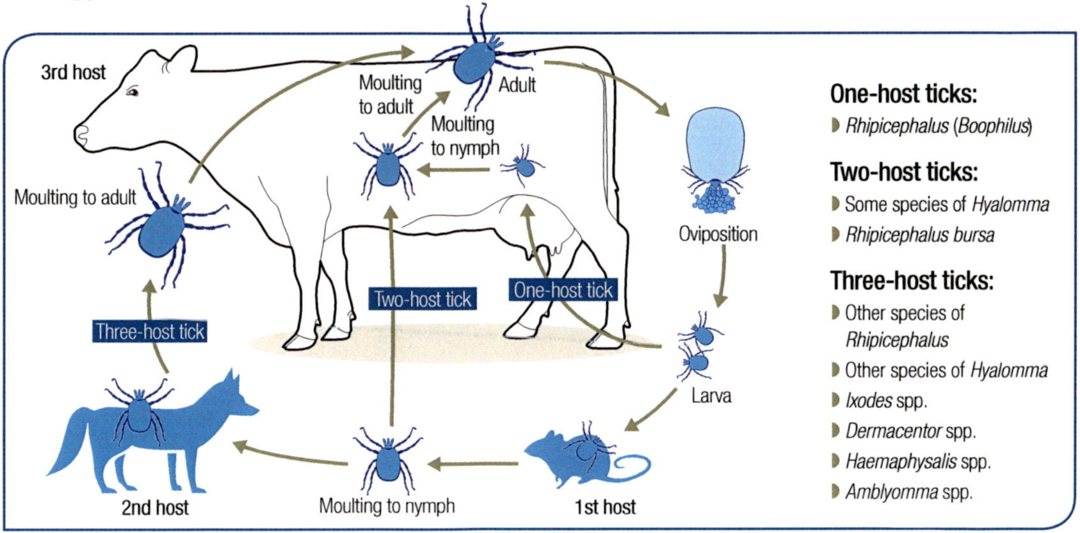

Figure 66. Most species of hard ticks have a three-host cycle, which explains why their control is so complicated.

Pathogenesis

- Traumatic action:
  - Inflammation and erythema.
  - Pruritus.
  - Wounds: infection/myiases.
- Depriving action:
  - Blood feeding.
- Disease vector:
  - Parasites (*Babesia*, *Theileria*, etc.).
  - Bacteria (*Borrelia, Coxiella, Rickettsia, Anaplasma*, etc.).
  - Viruses (*Flavivirus*, etc.).
- Toxic action (some species):
  - Neurotoxin: flaccid paralysis.

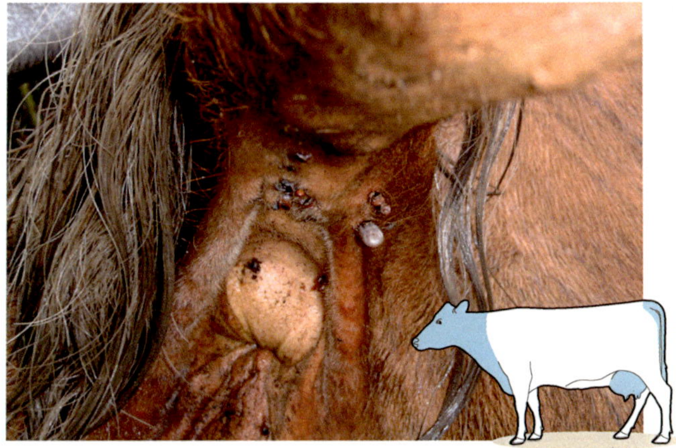

Figure 67. Ticks are easy to detect on the animal, generally at their preferred sites for attachment, such as the ears, face, neck, skin folds of the perineal and inguinal regions and under the tail.

Control

On the animal

- Manual removal.
- Acaricidal treatment (higher-risk periods).

On the environment

- Controlled burning of highly infested fields.
- Turn over the soil.
- Acaricide treatments.

- Avoid going out to pasture/outdoor the periods during which ticks are more active.
- Obtain information about the endemic species.

Figure 68. Tick control is usually based on measures applied to the animal, since most tick species use several hosts, which include wild animals.

Mange mite and lice infestation

Biology

Length of life cycle: 2-3 weeks

Mange mites:

- *Sarcoptes scabiei bovis*
- *Psoroptes equi bovis*
- *Chorioptes bovis*
- *Demodex bovis*

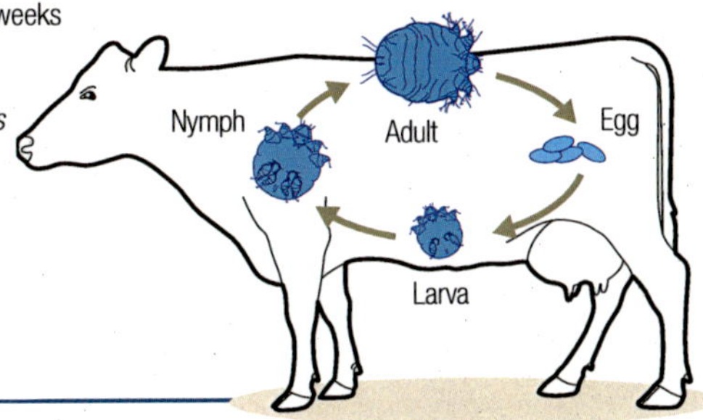

Length of life cycle: 3-4 weeks

Sucking lice:

- *Linognathus vituli*
- *Haematopinus eurysternus*
- *Solenopotes capillatus*

Chewing lice:

- *Bovicola bovis*

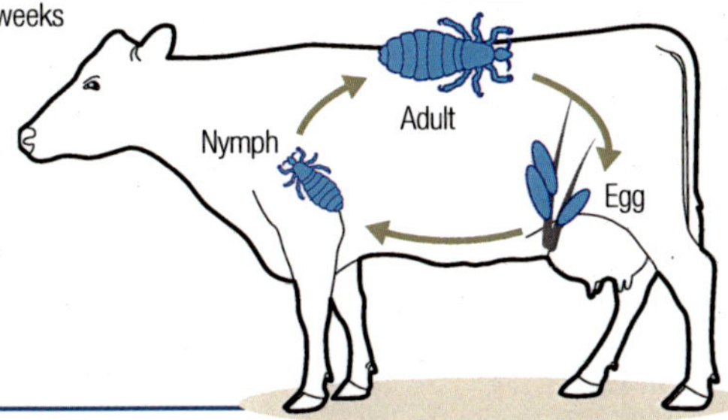

Figure 69. Both mange mites and lice complete their life cycle in the same animal. They only survive in the environment for a short period of time.

Sarcoptic mange

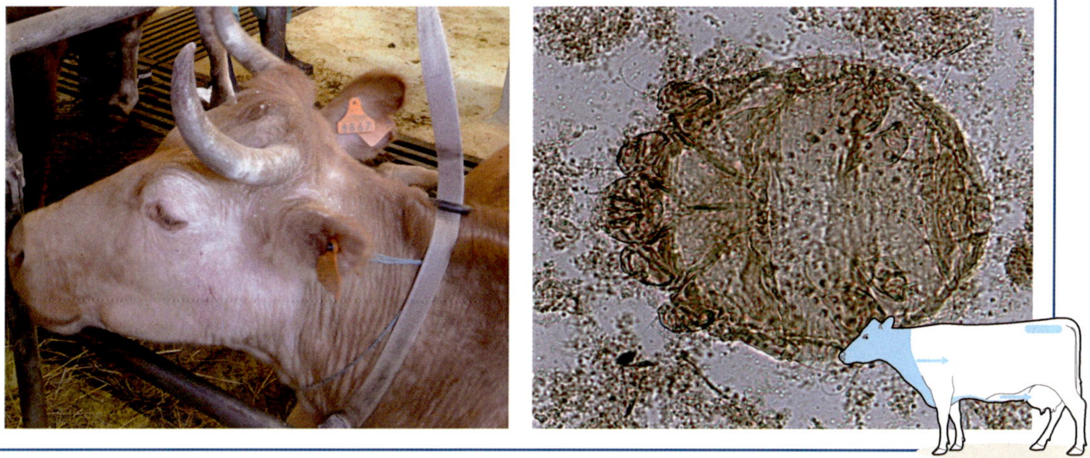

Figure 70. Sarcoptic mange is highly pruriginous, and is usually located on the head and neck, giving rise to characteristic skin folds. The animals should be handled with caution, as it is a zoonosis.

Psoroptic mange

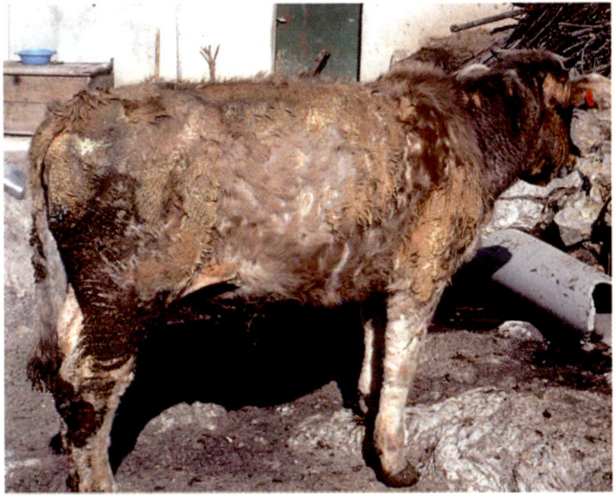

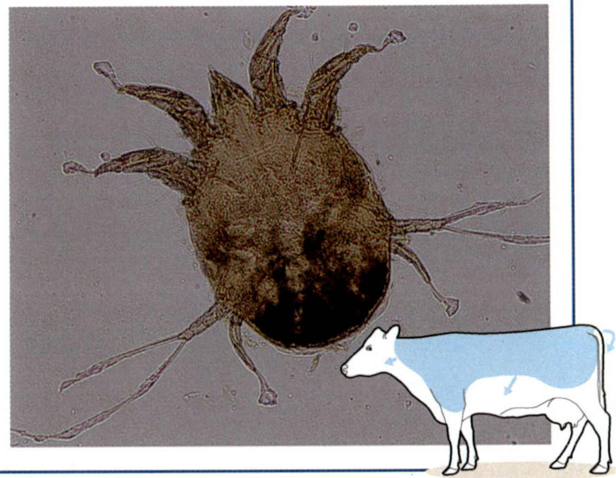

Figure 71. Psoroptic mange is also pruriginous, and affects areas of dense hair, such as the animal's back. If left untreated it may become generalised and extend to the whole body. Image courtesy of Dr. Pablo Díez Baños.

Chorioptic mange

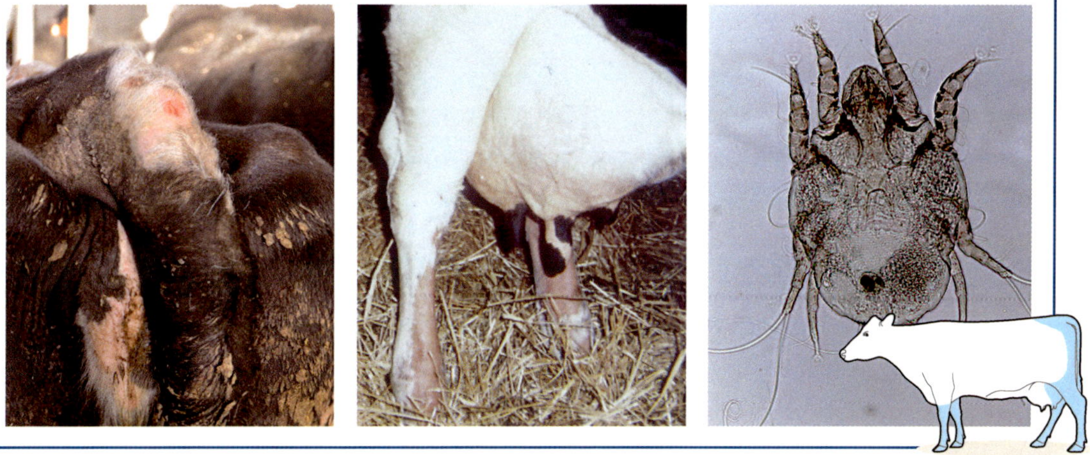

Figure 72. Chorioptic mange is the most frequent and least pruriginous type of mange. It usually appears at the base of the tail, on the inner thighs and legs. Image courtesy of Dr. Pablo Díez Baños.

Pediculosis

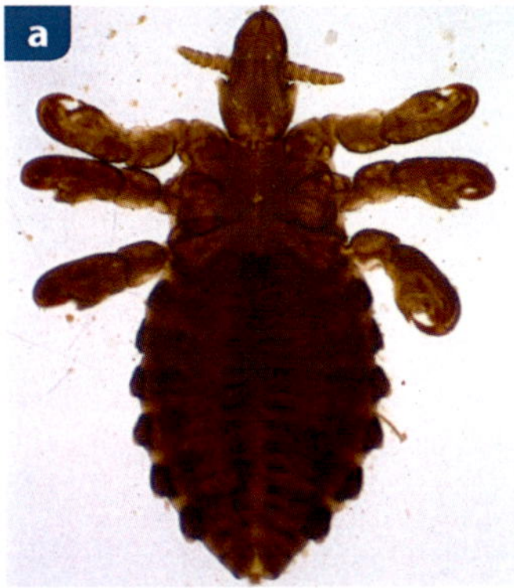

Haematopinus eurysternus

- Short-nosed cattle louse.
- Head narrower than the thorax.
- Blood-feeding lice.

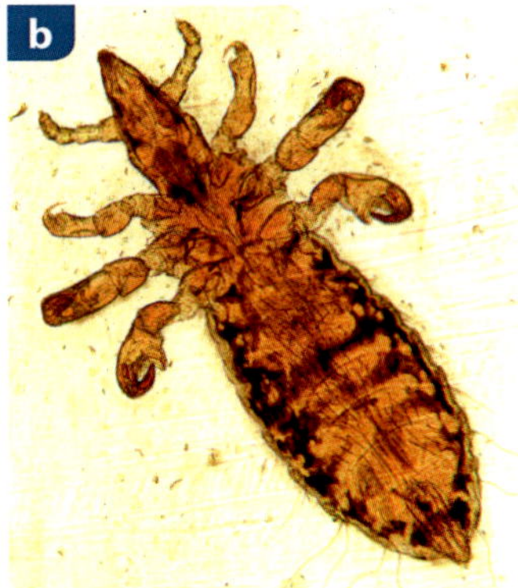

Linognathus vituli

- Long-nosed cattle louse.
- Head narrower than the thorax.
- Blood-feeding lice.

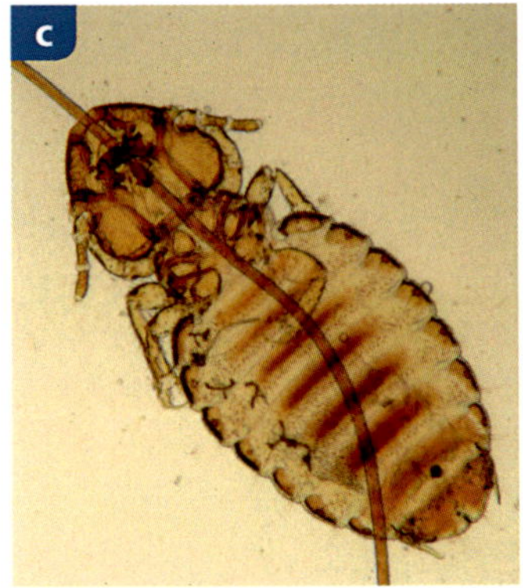

Bovicola bovis

- Head wider than the thorax.
- Feed on skin flakes.

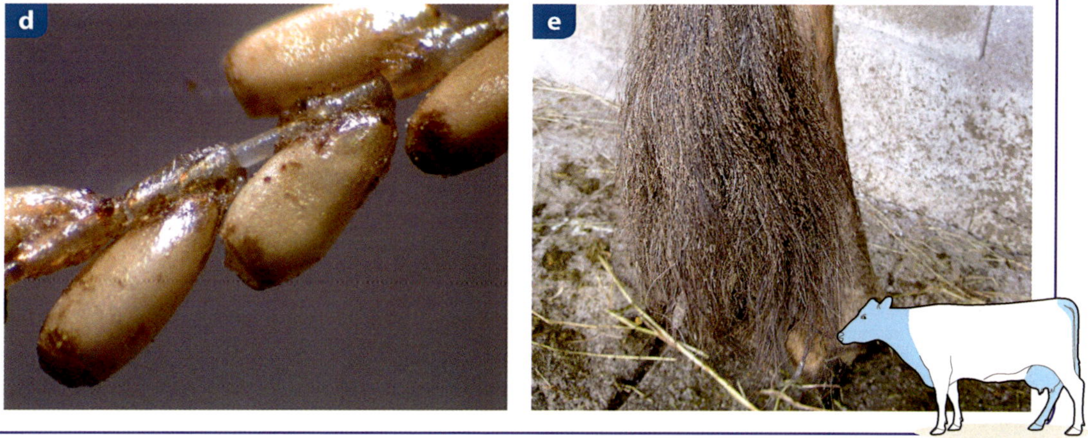

Figure 73. There are two types of lice: (a and b) Anoplura or sucking lice and (c) Mallophaga or chewing lice. Their eggs or (d and e) nits are usually located in specific areas and are easy to identify.

Diagnosis

Epidemiological suspicion

- High infectivity.
- Time of the year (autumn-winter).
- Pruritus.
- Alopecia, scabs, etc.
- Location of the lesions.

→ **Laboratory analysis**

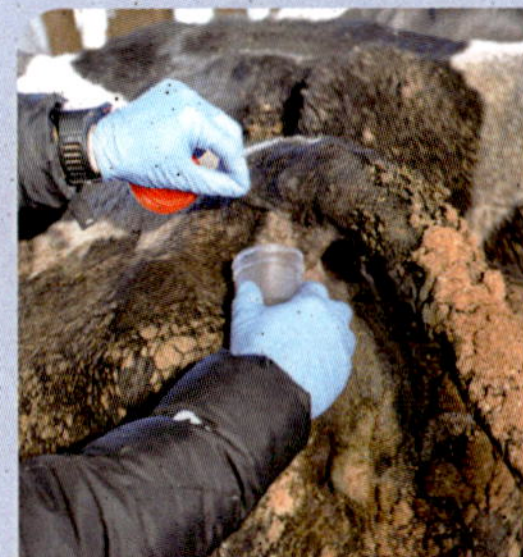

Mange

- **Scraping** on the edge of the lesions (deep: *Sarcoptes*):
  - Direct microscopic observation (*Psoroptes - Chorioptes*).
  - Observation after digestion of scabs with KOH at 10 % (all the genera).
- **ELISA test** (*Sarcoptes* spp.).

Lice

- Direct collection.
- Brushing.
- Microscopic identification of adults-nits.

Control

On the environment

- Cleaning and disinfection of the facilities, equipment, fixtures, etc.

On the animal

- Strategic treatment with acaricides/insecticides.
- Repeat the treatment at a 10- to 20-day interval: these drugs do not have an ovicidal action.
- Respect the quarantine period when bringing new animals into the herd.
- Appropriate diet.

Dictyocaulosis

Dictyocaulus viviparus

- Mainly affects young individuals.
- Clinical signs:
  - **Cough.**
  - **Tachypnoea/dyspnoea.**
  - **Crackles/stertor.**
  - Anorexia.
  - Poor overall condition.
- Diagnosis: coprological-immunological.
- Differential diagnosis: pasteurellosis, tuberculosis, BVD, IBR, etc.

a b

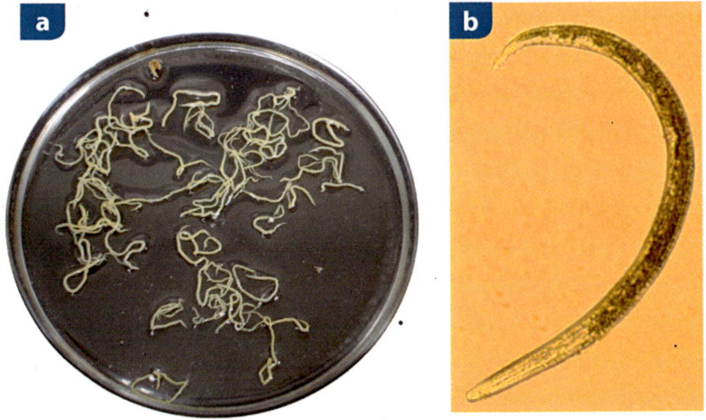

Figure 74. (a) The adults of *Dictyocaulus* are found in the trachea and bronchi and may reach 7 cm in length. (b) First-stage larvae can be identified by means of a coprological analysis.

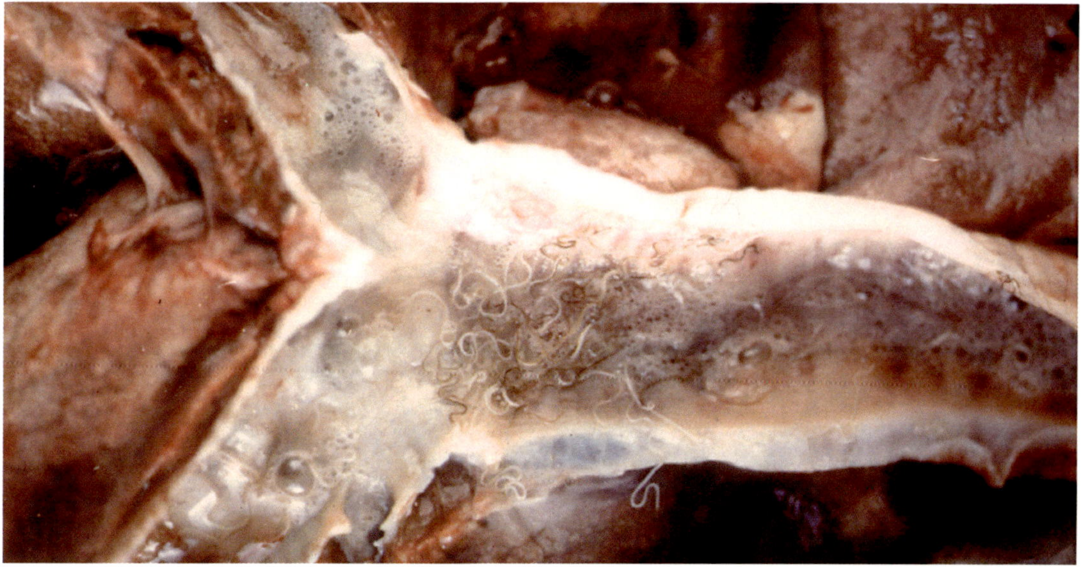

Figure 75. The irritating action of the adults of *D. viviparus* causes bronchitis and pneumonia. Image courtesy of Dr. Natividad Díez Baños.

Cysticercosis

Cysticercus bovis → *Taenia saginata*

- Location in muscles (tongue, masseters, myocardium, etc.).
- Definitive host: humans.

Cysticercus tenuicollis → *Taenia hydatigena*

- Location in liver, peritoneum.
- Definitive host: dog.

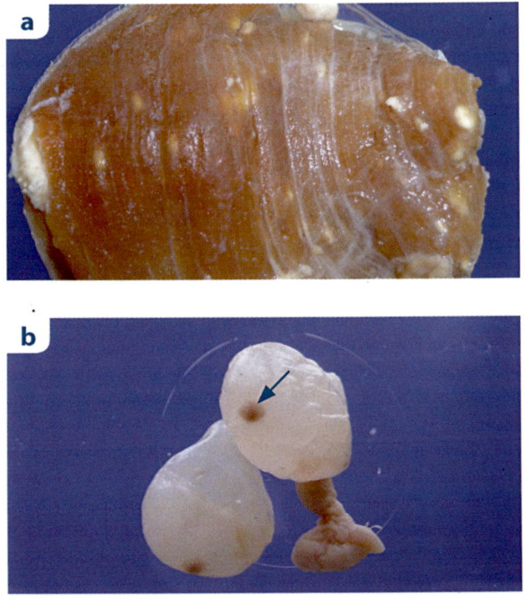

Figure 76. *Cysticercus* larvae contain only one protoscolex (arrow), which will give rise to a single adult cestode in the definitive host. Images courtesy of Dr. Ceferino López.

Hydatidosis

Hydatid cyst → *Echinococcus granulosus*

- Most affected organs:
  - Liver.
  - Lung.
- Definitive hosts: canids.

Cysticercosis and hydatidosis do not usually cause clinical signs and are therefore observed at slaughter. The affected organs are always condemned.

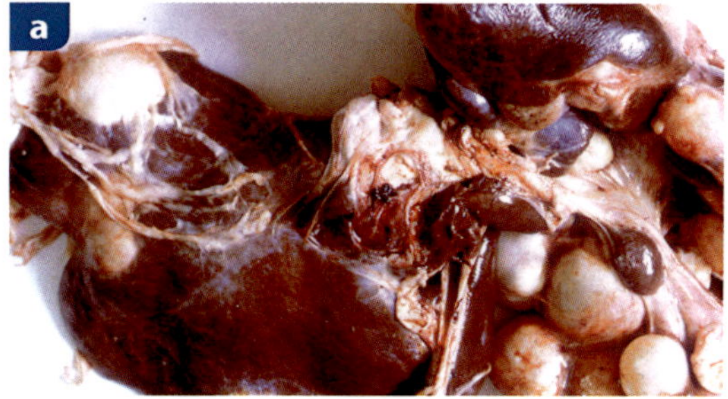

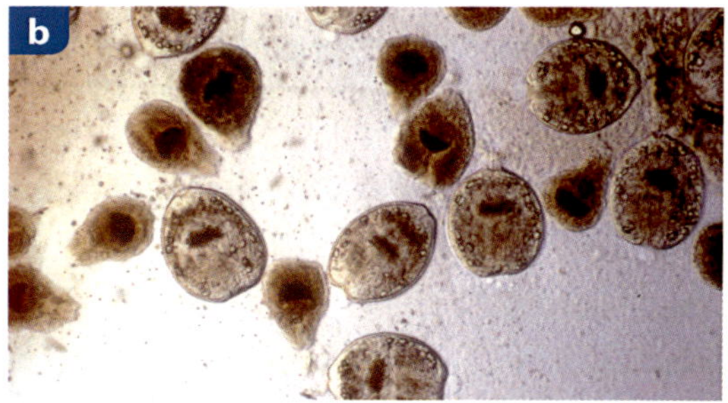

Figure 77. (a) Hydatid cysts contain a high amount of (b) protoscoleces and will thus give rise to hundreds of adult cestodes in the definitive host. Images courtesy of Dr. Caridad Sánchez-Acedo.

Clinical-epidemiological diagnosis

- Presumptive.
- Must be confirmed with laboratory results.

Clinical diagnosis

- General clinical signs: abortions, anaemia, weakness, apathy, loss of weight, etc.
- Local clinical signs: digestive, respiratory, cutaneous signs, etc.

Epidemiological diagnosis

- Age, sex and breed.
- Spread: percentage of sick animals, other species affected, etc.
- Management: rearing system, stress factors, housing, nutrition, etc.
- Weather conditions.

Diagnostic parasitology methods

Direct diagnosis

Its purpose is to detect the parasite, one of its stages or constituting parts (DNA, antigens, etc.):

- Coprological diagnosis.
- Haematological diagnosis.
- Dermatological diagnosis.
- Histological, histopathological and pathological diagnosis.
- Immunological diagnosis.
- Molecular diagnosis.

Indirect diagnosis

It assesses the damage caused by the parasite or parameters related to the host's response against the parasitic infection:

- Immunological diagnosis.
- Methods evaluating plasma parameters.
- Histopathological and pathological diagnosis.

Coprological diagnosis

Collection of faecal samples

Directly from the rectum or recently excreted faeces

Label and refrigerate samples (preserves and slows down parasite development)

Table 3. Techniques used to detect parasitic forms in faeces.

Gross examination	▸ Presence of macroscopic parasites (adults, larvae...). ▸ Presence of blood, mucus, etc.
Microscopic examination	**Direct smear** ▸ Fast but low sensitivity. ▸ Can be performed on the farm. ▸ Complement with other tests. ▸ Smear staining can detect *Cryptosporidium* oocysts.

Microscopic examination	Concentration techniques (higher sensitivity)	**Migration** ▸ The Baermann apparatus is used. ▸ To detect larvae of bronchopulmonary nematodes.	
		Sedimentation ▸ Used for forms with high densities, which do not float in the most commonly used floating solutions. ▸ Identification of eggs.	**McMaster method** ▸ For parasite quantification. ▸ Use a McMaster chamber. ▸ Knowing the initial amount of faeces is necessary.
		Flotation ▸ Concentrates the parasites using high-density solutions (p >1.20). ▸ Saturated salt solution, sugar flotation solution, $ZnSO_4$, etc. ▸ Cestode and nematode eggs, protozoan cysts and oocysts.	
		Identification of third-stage larvae of gastrointestinal nematodes (strongylids) ▸ After confirmation of the presence of gastrointestinal nematode eggs by means of flotation. ▸ To identify the genera involved. ▸ Perform a coproculture to obtain third-stage larvae.	

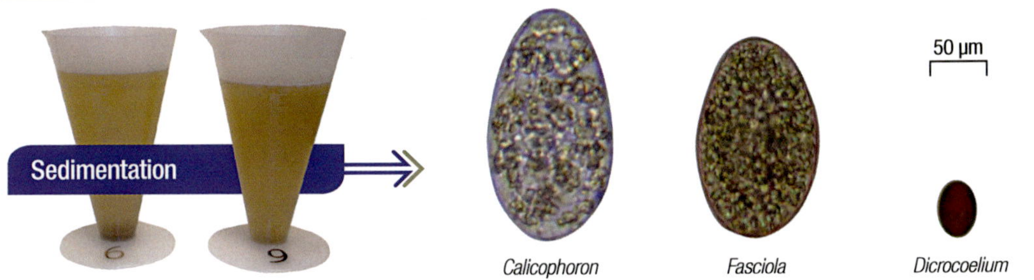
Sedimentation
6
9
50 µm
Calicophoron
Fasciola
Dicrocoelium

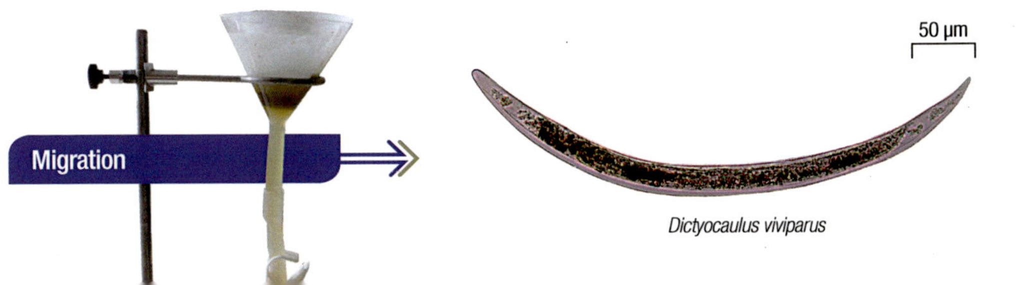
Migration
50 µm
Dictyocaulus viviparus

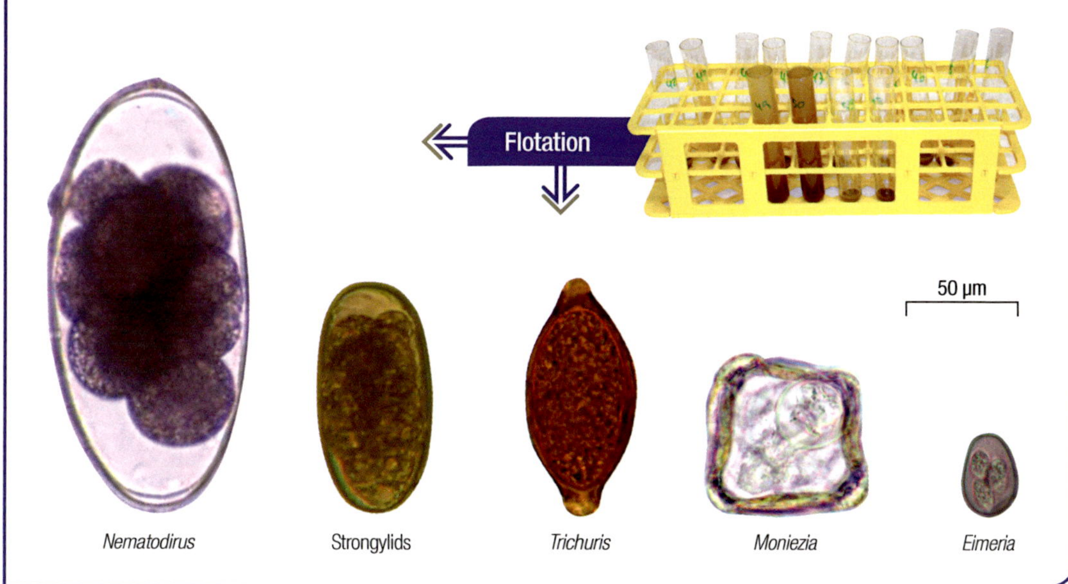

Figure 78. Main coprological techniques and parasites most frequently identified in cattle.

Table 4. Measurement ranges of eggs/oocysts of the most common parasites in cattle (Thienpont et al., 1986).

Parasites	Length (μ)	Width (μ)
Fasciola	130-145	70-90
Calicophoron	125-180	73-103
Dicrocoelium	38-45	22-30
Nematodirus	130-260	67-121
Trichuris	70-80	30-42
Strongylids	62-125	29-59
Moniezia	80-90	80-90
Dictyocaulus viviparus	390-450	25
Eimeria	10-40	10-30

Table 5. Considerations to bear in mind when carrying out a coprological analysis.

Advantages	Shortcomings
▸ Used to identify parasitic forms directly. ▸ Economical, simple and relatively rapid. ▸ Parasitic forms can be identified. Useful to assess treatment efficacy. ▸ The farm's health status can be assessed in an economical manner with pools (mix of faeces from several individuals).	▸ Low sensitivity: low-intensity parasitic infections or during the prepatent period. ▸ Experienced personnel required. Not useful for field diagnosis. ▸ Counts are indicative; the parasitic load cannot be estimated with accuracy. ▸ Sensitivity with pools is lower than when individual samples are collected.

Haematological diagnosis

- Whole blood samples must be used: tubes with an anticoagulant, preferably EDTA.
- A rapid processing prevents sample deterioration and RBC deformation.
- Thin blood smear is the technique most commonly used:
  - It should be analysed by personnel with experience in the identification of parasitic forms found in blood.
  - Quick staining can be performed in only three steps with some commercial kits.
- A drop of fresh blood (direct smear method) may also be examined for the diagnosis of *Trypanosoma* spp., as the movement of trypomastigotes can be detected.

Dermatological diagnosis

- In flea, lice or tick infestations, the parasite can be identified directly on the animal.
- In cases of mange, skin scrapings should be carried out to collect scabs and mites:
  - They should be performed at the transition between the affected tissue and the healthy tissue, over a 6-8 cm^2 surface.
  - If *Sarcoptes* spp. is suspected, the scraping should be deeper; for *Demodex* spp., hairs should be pulled out with their follicles.
  - Identification is made easier by adding KOH at 10 %, which breaks up tissues and releases potential mites.

Histological, histopathological and pathological diagnosis

- Used to detect the parasite in organs or tissue samples.
- Some lesions or histological abnormalities may be indirectly associated with the presence of a specific parasite.
- They are usually post-mortem techniques, although biopsy samples may also be used.

Diagnosis of plasma parameters

- Parameters related to a general response of the host against the parasite are usually used:
  - Eosinophilia.
  - Increased liver enzyme levels (GLDH and γ-GT...).
- The level of some substances (serum pepsinogen) is increased as a consequence of the parasite's action.

Immunological methods

- Indirect: to detect the immune response (antibodies) against the parasite, especially in serum or milk.
- Direct: to recognise parasite antigens in both serum and faeces (coproantigens).
- Knowing the antibody concentration (serum antibody titre) is sometimes useful.
- Enzyme immunoassays (ELISA), complement fixation (CF), immunofluorescence (IF), indirect agglutination (IA), Western blot (EITB) and immunohistochemistry (IHC) are among the most common techniques.

Table 6. Considerations to bear in mind when performing immunological techniques.

Advantages	Shortcomings
• High sensitivity, specificity and reproducibility. • Rapid. • Low cost. • Diagnosis of infections with parasites that are not located in the digestive or respiratory system. • Early detection: parasitic infections can be detected during the prepatent period. • Possible to differentiate between acute and chronic infections. • Can be automated.	• Difficult to obtain antigens and monoclonal antibodies. • Recent studies cannot be differentiated from previous ones or the efficacy of treatments assessed due to the persistence of antibodies. • The presence of antibodies cannot be correlated with active infection; it only indicates exposure to the parasite. • Possible non-specific or crossed reactions between similar parasite families.

Molecular techniques

Table 7. Considerations to bear in mind when performing molecular techniques.

Advantages	Shortcomings
▸ High sensitivity and specificity. ▸ A small sample is required. ▸ Dead animals can be processed. ▸ Possible to differentiate between different varieties of the same species and their zoonotic potential. ▸ Possible to quantify the presence of the parasite with the qPCR technique. ▸ Very useful in taxonomic and epidemiological studies or in eradication programmes.	▸ Not possible to differentiate between DNA from live parasites and DNA from dead parasites. ▸ Not available for daily use. ▸ Does not detect mixed infections. ▸ Expensive.

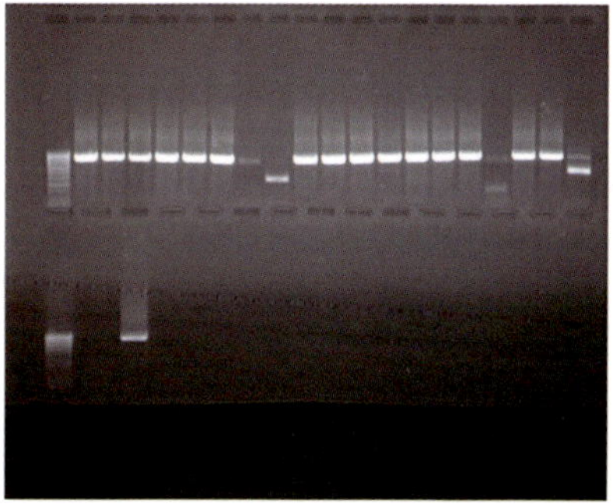

Figure 79. PCR.

Table 8. Main anthelmintic drugs authorised for use in cattle in Europe.

Active ingredient	Dose (mg/kg body weight)	Route of administration	Use in lactating animals*	Cestodes	Trematodes				Nematodes				Comments
				Moniezia	Immature *Fasciola*	Adult *Fasciola*	*Dicrocoelium*	Rumen flukes	Strongylids	*Nematodirus*	*Trichuris*	*Dictyocaulus*	
Doramectin	0.2	s.c.	✗						+	+	+	+	
Eprinomectin	0.5	Pour-on	✓						+	+	+	+	0 days in milk
Ivermectin	0.2 0.5	s.c. Pour-on	✗ ✗						+ +	+ +	+ +	+ +	
Moxidectin	0.2-1 0.5	s.c. Pour-on	✗ ✓						+ +	+ +	+	+ +	
Netobimin	7.5-20	p.o.	✓	+		+			+	+	+	+	Effective against *Fasciola* at 20 mg/kg
Triclabendazole	12 20	p.o. Pour-on	✗ ✗		+	+							
Albendazole	7.5-10	p.o.	✓	+		+	+		+	+		+	Effective against *Fasciola* at 10 mg/kg
Fenbendazole	7.5	p.o.	✓						+	+		+	
Oxfendazole	4.5-5	p.o.	✗	+					+	+	+	+	

Active ingredient	Dose (mg/kg body weight)	Route of administration	Use in lactating animals*	Cestodes	Trematodes				Nematodes				Comments
				Moniezia	Immature *Fasciola*	Adult *Fasciola*	*Dicrocoelium*	Rumen flukes	Strongylids	*Nematodirus*	*Trichuris*	*Dictyocaulus*	
Levamisole	7.5	p.o., s.c.	✗						+	+		+	
Clorsulon	2 7	s.c. p.o.	✗ ✗			+							
Nitroxynil	10	s.c.	✗		+/-	+			+				Immature *Fasciola* >6 weeks
Closantel	2.5 20	p.o. Pour-on	✗ ✗		+/-	+		+	+				Immature *Fasciola* >6 weeks
Oxyclozanide	10-15	p.o.	✓	+		+		+					Can be used in milk if the product contains no other antiparasitic drug

* Their use is not permitted in cattle producing milk for human consumption, including during the dry period. All anthelmintics have a withdrawal period of 3 days in milk (on average), except eprinomectin.

The dosages and withdrawal periods or restrictions on use must be checked according to the manufacturer of the product to be used and the legislation in force in each region/country.

Table 9. Main endo/ecto parasiticides with activity against protozoa, insects and mites and authorised for use in cattle in Europe.

Active ingredient	Dose (mg/kg body weight)	Route of administration	Protozoa				Arthropods							Comments
			Babesia	*Theileria*	*Cryptosporidium*	*Eimeria*	*Sarcoptes*	*Psoroptes*	*Chorioptes*	Sucking lice	Chewing lice	Ticks	*Hypoderma*	
Doramectin	0.2	s.c.					+	+	+/-	+	+/-	+/-	+	
Eprinomectin	0.5	Pour-on					+		+	+	+		+	0 days in milk
Ivermectin	0.2 0.5	s.c. Pour-on					+ +	+	+/- +/-	+ +	+/- +		+ +	
Moxidectin	0.2-0.5	s.c. Pour-on					+ +	+ +	+/- +	+ +	+/- +		+ +	
Closantel	5 20	p.o. Pour-on											+/-	Effective only against second and third instars of *Hypoderma*
Cypermethrin	Variable depending on use and manufacturer	Pour-on Topical								+ +	+ +	 +		
Deltamethrin	0.3-1.2	Pour-on								+	+	+		

Active ingredient	Dose (mg/kg body weight)	Route of administration	Protozoa				Arthropods							Comments
			Babesia	*Theileria*	*Cryptosporidium*	*Eimeria*	*Sarcoptes*	*Psoroptes*	*Chorioptes*	Sucking lice	Chewing lice	Ticks	*Hypoderma*	
Decoquinate	1	p.o.				+								
Sulfadimidine	166	p.o.				+								
Diclazuril	1	p.o.				+								
Toltrazuril	15	p.o.				+								
Imidocarb	1-2	s.c.	+											
Tetracyclines	10-20	i.m./s.c.		+										
Halofuginone	0.1	p.o.			+									7 consecutive days

The dosages and withdrawal periods or restrictions on use must be checked according to the manufacturer of the product to be used and the legislation in force in each region/country.

Anthelmintic resistance

- Capacity of a population of parasites to tolerate doses of a drug that are effective against a normal population.
- This problem is increasing, especially in other species, such as sheep. Detected in *Fasciola hepatica*, strongylids, mange mites, etc.
- It appears due to:
  - Continuous and reiterated use of anthelmintics, especially of drugs with the same mechanism of action.
  - Poor use of anthelmintics (wrong calculation of the dose, etc.), which results in subdosing.
  - Diagnostic errors.
- How to reduce the appearance of anthelmintic resistance:
  - Previous aetiological diagnosis.
  - Correct calculation of the dose.
  - Rotation of anthelmintics between the different families.

References

Almería, S., Lopez-Gatius, F. 2013. Bovine neosporosis: Clinical and practical aspects. *Research in Veterinary Science*, 95: 303-309.

Alvarez-García, G., Frey, C.F., Mora, L.M., Schares, G. 2013. A century of bovine besnoitiosis: an unknown disease re-emerging in Europe. *Trends in Parasitology.* Aug; 29(8): 407-415.

Arias, M.S., Sanchís, J., Francisco, I., Francisco, R., Piñeiro, P., Cazapal-Monteiro, C., Cortiñas, F.J., Suárez, J.L., Sánchez-Andrade, R., Paz-Silva, A. 2013. The efficacy of four anthelmintics against *Calicophoron daubneyi* in naturally infected dairy cattle. *Veterinary Parasitology*, 197(1-2): 126-129.

Arias, M.S., Súarez, J., Cortiñas, F.J., Francisco, I., Súarez, J.L., Romasanta, A., Cazapal-Monteiro, C., Sánchez-Andrade, R., Paz-Silva, A. 2012. Restoration of fungal biota in the soil is essential to prevent infection by endoparasites in grazing animals. In: Fungi: Types, Environmental Impact and Role in Disease. A. Paz-Silva and M.S. Arias, Ed. Hauppauge, NY: Nova Science Publishers, USA; 341-358.

Bishop, R., Musoke, A., Morzaria, S., Gardner, M., Nene, V. 2004. *Theileria*: intracellular protozoan parasites of wild and domestic ruminants transmitted by ixodid ticks. *Parasitology*, 129, S271–S283.

Bock, R., Jackson, I., Vos, A.D., Jorgensen, W. 2004. Babesiosis of cattle. *Parasitology*, 129: 247-269.

Bowman, D.D. Georgis' Parasitology for Veterinarians, 10th Ed. Saunders, 2013.

Cortinas, R., Jones, C.J. 2006. Ectoparasites of cattle and small ruminants. *Veterinary Clinics of North America: Food Animal Practice.* Nov; 22(3): 673-693.

Dakkak, A. 2010. Echinococcosis/hydatidosis: a severe threat in Mediterranean countries. *Veterinary Parasitology.* Nov; 24; 174(1-2): 2-11.

Dalton, J.P. Fasciolosis. CAB International Publishing. Wallingford, Oxon, UK, 1999.

Daugschies, A., Najdrowski, M. 2005. Eimeriosis in cattle: current understanding. *Journal of Veterinary Medicine. B, Infectious Diseases and Veterinary Public Health.* Dec; 52(10): 417-427.

Dubey, J.P., Schares, G., Ortega-Mora, L.M. 2007. Epidemiology and Control of Neosporosis and *Neospora caninum. Clinical Microbiology Reviews,* 20(2): 323-367.

Fayer, R., Xiao, L. *Cryptosporidium* and cryptosporidiosis. 2nd Ed. CRC Press, Boca Raton, Florida, 2008.

Food and Agriculture Organization of the United Nations. Manual for the Recognition of Exotic Diseases of Livestock. Retrieved from http://www.spc.int

Hendrix, C.M. Diagnóstico parasitológico veterinario. Ed. Harcourt Brace, 1999.

Hendrix, C.M., Robinson, E. Diagnostic Parasitology for Veterinary Technicians, 4th Ed. Mosby, 2011.

Kahn, C.M., Line, S., editors. The Merck veterinary manual [online]. Whitehouse Station, NJ: Merck and Co., 2006.

L'Hostis, M., Seegers, H. 2002. Tick-borne parasitic diseases in cattle: current knowledge and prospective risk analysis related to the ongoing evolution in French cattle farming systems. *Veterinary Research,* 33: 599-611.

MAFF (Ministry of Agriculture, Fisheries and Food). Manual of veterinary parasitological laboratory techniques. H.M.S.O. London, 1986.

Melhorn, H., Düwell, D., Raether, W. Atlas of Veterinary Parasitology. Grass. Barcelona, Spain, 1992.

Mosqueda, J., Olvera-Ramírez, A., Aguilar-Tipacamú, G., Cantó, G.J. 2012. Current Advances in Detection and Treatment of Babesiosis. *Current Medicinal Chemistry,* 19(10): 1504-1518.

O'Handley, R.M., Olson, M.E. 2006. Giardiasis and cryptosporidiosis in ruminants. *Veterinary Clinics of North America: Food Animal Practice.* Nov; 22(3): 623-643.

Panuska, C. 2006. Lungworms of ruminants. *Veterinary Clinics of North America: Food Animal Practice.* Nov; 22(3): 583-593.

Kaufmann, J. Parasitic Infections of Domestic Animals. A diagnostic manual. Basel, Switzerland: Birkhauser Verlag, 1996.

Paz-Silva, A., Arias, M., Francisco, I., Cortiñas, F.J., Francisco, R., Díaz, P., Suárez, J.L., Díez-Baños, P., Morrondo, P., Sánchez-Andrade, R. 2010. Cross-immunity and interpretation of the diagnosis of parasitic trematodosis in ruminants by means of immunoenzymatic probes. In: Veterinary Parasitology. G.V. LaMann (Ed). NY, Nova Science Publishers, Inc; 271-288.

Ploeger, H.W. 2002. *Dictyocaulus viviparus*: re-emerging or never been away? *Trends in Parasitology.* Aug; 18(8): 329-332.

Sirois, M. Laboratory Manual for Laboratory Procedures for Veterinary Technicians, 6th Ed. Mosby, 2014.

Taira, N., Ando, Y., Williams, J.C. A color atlas of Clinical Helminthology of domestic animals. Chiskusan Publishing Company, Tokyo, 2003.

Taylor, M.A., Coop, R.L., Wall, R.L. Veterinary Parasitology, 3rd Ed. Wiley-Blackwell, 2007.

Thienpont, D., Rochette, F., Vanparijs, O.F.J. Diagnosing Helminthiasis By Coprological Examination. Janssen Research Foundation; Beerse, Belgium, 1986.

Uilenberg, G. 2006. *Babesia*-A historical overview. *Veterinary Parasitology,* 138: 3-10.

Urquhart, G.M., Armour, J., Duncan, J.L., Jennings, F.W., Dunn, A.M. Veterinary Parasitology. 2nd Ed. Longman Higher Education, 1996.

Wall, R., Shearer, D. Veterinary Ectoparasites: Biology, Pathology and Control. 2nd Ed. Wiley-Blackwell, 2001.

World Organization for Animal Health (OIE). Retrieved from http://www.oie.int